Enter the Sensuous
Realm of Scents

Fragrance, undulating through the atmosphere like a perfumed veil of Aphrodite, is one of life's most lovely gifts for the sensuous woman. Mysterious and mystical, fragrance stirs deep pools of pure sensation. Like a winged messenger from another kingdom, scent whispers an unspoken seduction that liberates emotion, unleashes memory, and excites true pleasure in its delightful embrace.

This phenomenon of fragrance, quintessential and ungraspable, has for millennia been miraculously captured in its most elemental state. Through various processes to extract the highly volatile aromatic oil from its secret recesses within the plant, pure fragrance—the essence of the flower—may be contained like a genie in a jar.

These essential oils—the jasmine with which Cleopatra drenched the sails of her barge in expectation of Mark Antony, the rose oil favored by Caesar's faithful wife—may be used by the woman of today to awaken her sensuality and passion for living in the here and now. Experience the delightful enchantments of the essential oils and become a wise enchantress through the gentle sorcery of scent.

About the Author

Elisabeth Millar is a native New Yorker now living in Brighton, England, with her husband and son. A former medical writer and editor of several scientific journals, as well as the creative director for an international pharmaceutical marketing firm, she currently focuses on ways women can find pleasure in the everyday joys of living. With aromatherapist Ann Woodhead, she runs a fragrance consultancy called Fragrant Veil that creates personalized fragrances for women. She is also the cofounder of the Novalis School for Spiritual Development in Brighton.

To Write to the Author

If you wish to contact the author or would like more information about this book, please write to the author in care of Llewellyn Worldwide and we will forward your request. Both the author and publisher appreciate hearing from you and learning of your enjoyment of this book and how it has helped you. Llewellyn Worldwide cannot guarantee that every letter written to the author can be answered, but all will be forwarded. Please write to:

Elisabeth Millar
℅ Llewellyn Worldwide
P.O. Box 64383, Dept. 1-56718-491-X
St. Paul, MN 55164-0383, U.S.A.

Please enclose a self-addressed stamped envelope for reply, or $1.00 to cover costs. If outside U.S.A., enclose international postal reply coupon.

Many of Llewellyn's authors have websites with additional information and resources. For more information, please visit our website at:

http://www.llewellyn.com

The Fragrant Veil

Scents for the Sensuous Woman

Elisabeth Millar

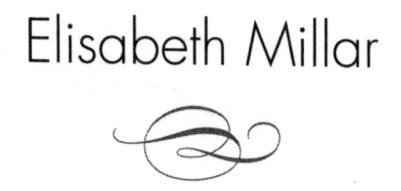

2000
Llewellyn Publications
St. Paul, Minnesota 55164-0383, U.S.A.

First Edition
First Printing, 2000

Book design and editing by Rebecca Zins
Cover design by Anne Marie Garrison
Oil blends created by Ann Woodhead,
  Fragrance Consultant

Library of Congress Cataloging-in-Publication Data
Millar, Elisabeth.
   The fragrant veil: scents for the sensuous woman /
Elisabeth Millar. — 1st ed.
   p.   cm.
   ISBN 1-56718-491-X
   1. Essences and essential oils. 2. Beauty, Personal.

GT2340 .F73 2000
391.6'3 — dc21
                                          00-055794

Disclaimer: These recipes have not been tested by the publisher. Personal sensitivities to ingredients should be researched before using them.

Llewellyn Worldwide does not participate in, endorse, or have any authority or responsibility concerning private business transactions between our authors and the public.
   All mail addressed to the author is forwarded but the publisher cannot, unless specifically instructed by the author, give out an address or phone number.

Llewellyn Publications
A Division of Llewellyn Worldwide, Ltd.
P.O. Box 64383, Dept. 1-56718-491-X
St. Paul, MN 55164-0383, U.S.A.
www.llewellyn.com

Printed in the United States of America
on recycled paper

To my parents
Lore and Joseph Kosh
with love and gratitude

Contents

Acknowledgments

to my beloved husband, Joe Eagle,
for his enduring love and support;
to my wise teachers,
Christina Sahin and Marilyn Curran;
to my agents at Paraview
and my publisher, Llewellyn,
for lifting the veil;
and to all those who
were so willing to help . . .
my deepest thanks

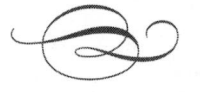

Special Thanks

to Ann Woodhead
for her help in the
creation of *The Fragrant Veil*
and the beautiful blends
it contains

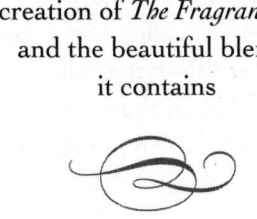

An Invitation . . .
For the Sensuous Woman

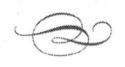

The sensuous woman stands still, silently caressing the moment with her attention. Receptive, aware, she stops in the now to savor its richness. Time, like a wide expanse, envelops her. She is enchanted, under a spell of the miraculous, filled with a sense of wonder. Aroused by beauty, moved by its poignancy, the sensuous woman embraces life, inviting it to enter like a lover into union—a marriage of one, unique Woman with all-mysterious Life, a marriage of earthly delights. This passionate sense of connection, this encompassing sensuality, celebrates life with mindfulness and joy.

Mindful of the shades of green in springtime, of sounds emerging from the stillness like melodies in the rustle of the wind, the sensuous woman reaches out to the world with her senses and through her senses receives its marvels. She tastes the sunshine on her lips and feels warm air like the breath of an angel on her face. She is sentient, sensitive, alive with perception. And here, fully in the present, she pauses to admire white roses pendulously overhanging a garden gate. She bends to deeply inhale their fragrance bursting from velvet petals. The scent captures her, wrapping her in a veil of fragrance, and she smiles.

Fragrance, ethereal and sublime as the soul of a flower, penetrates her psyche, evoking deeply pleasurable emotions through the sensual sense of smell. More quickly transmitted than sensation, more precisely recorded than sound, more permanently stored than visual memory, scent communicates directly with the oldest and most primal part of the brain. And in this ancient seat of the mind, responsible for all emotion and memory, all primordial drives and functions of survival, all intuitive knowing and all intimations of the unknowable, fragrance sparks the very source of joy.

Joyously surrendering to the magic of the moment, surrounded by the scent of roses, the sensuous woman opens to the wisdom of the flower so flawlessly articulated in the metaphor of fragrance. A crescendo of emotions cascades through her and—in an instant of perfect merging—the woman, inspired by the gently yielding feminine fragrance of the rose, feels love.

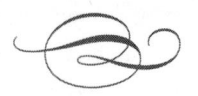

A love affair between the senses and the great suitor Life—an intimate relationship with living—awaits every woman who in her wisdom chooses to fill her heart with the multitude of wonders unfolding in the stillness of a moment. Of these wonders, fragrance—undulating through the atmosphere like a perfumed veil of Aphrodite—is one of life's most lovely gifts for the sensuous woman.

Mysterious and mystical—at once unseen and undeniable, silent though commanding, fleeting but never forgotten—fragrance stirs deep pools of pure sensation. Like a winged messenger from another kingdom, scent whispers an unspoken seduction that liberates emotion, unleashes memory, and excites true pleasure in its delightful embrace. A fragrant embrace so touching yet intangible, so understood yet undefinable, so elusive, so pervasive, so subtle, so provocative, fragrance is phenomenon—so other and so desired.

This phenomenon of fragrance, quintessential and ungraspable, has for millennia been miraculously captured in its most elemental state. Through various processes to extract the highly volatile aromatic oil from its secret recesses within the plant, pure fragrance—the essence of the flower—may be contained like a genie in a jar.

Holding within their molecules the mysteries of fragrance, the essential oils have been studied for at least 6,000 years in Egypt, Greece, and Rome. An unreproducible product of nature, essential oil was found to possess not only all the potentials and properties of its parent plant but also a unique personality, an individual charm that worked its special magic on the body, mind, and emotions of those who smelled its fragrance.

In antiquity, essential oils were used in all areas of daily life—as incense to inspire, as unguents to beautify, as perfumes to entice, as medicines to heal—as part of an exuberant sensuality and an extravagant thanksgiving to the gods. Often more valuable than gold, vast quantities of precious aromatics were burned on temple altars throughout the day. Statues of the holy were anointed with fragrant oil: myrrh for the moon god; frankincense for the sun. During religious festivals, fortunes from King Solomon's mines were consumed as incense continuously wafted through public buildings and city squares. On state occasions the streets were lined with flowers and fountains flowed with aromatic water. Honored guests at Roman feasts were misted with exotic scents, the wings of birds were tipped with aromatic oil to perfume the air, and slave girls danced with scented cones of oil on their heads that exuded fragrance in the sun. Food was flavored with violets and served on ornate earthenware soaked in fragrant oil; wine was seeped in roses. And the women, sensing the evocative powers of fragrance, adorned themselves in aromatics. Their baths were scented with lavender . . . their faces nourished with frankincense . . . their hair combed with cedarwood . . . their bodies perfumed for love with rose oil on the lips, jasmine on the nipples, and sandalwood on the thighs.

These essential oils—the jasmine with which Cleopatra drenched the sails of her barge in expectation of Mark Antony, the rose oil favored by Caesar's faithful wife—these same oils may be used by the woman of today to awaken and enhance a sensuous connection, a passion for living in the here and now.

The Fragrant Veil invites you to experience the delightful enchantments of the essential oils and to become a wise enchantress through the gentle sorcery of scent—an enchantress who neither tricks nor leads astray but rather guides through the mysterious powers of fragrance, a conscious process of mindfulness and a joyous celebration of the wonders within her, beside her, and around her.

Pure Fragrance
The Essential Oils of Nature

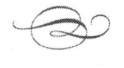

The fragrance of aromatic plants and trees is contained in minute droplets of a highly volatile oil called the essence of the plant. Produced and stored in tiny oil glands located throughout the plant—on the surface of a leaf, in the petals of a flower, the peel of a fruit, the roots, the resin, or the heartwood of a tree—the essence may be found in more than one location in the plant or may travel during its life cycle from one area to another. The amount of essence in a plant similarly varies from abundant to scarce depending on the species as well as the time of day or year. Composed of sometimes more than 100 constituents, each essence is a highly complex chemical structure that acts synergistically to regulate the plant's functioning, promote growth, protect against disease, and encourage fertilization.

The extracted fragrance is a non-greasy, highly volatile oil that, unlike fatty plant oils such as olive or sweet almond oil, readily disperses into the atmosphere. Borrowing from musical terminology, the oils are classified by their speed of evaporation from most rapid top notes to middle notes and most lingering base notes. These volatile oils, called either essential or, more generically, aromatic oils, powerfully affect the mind and emotions through the most sensual of senses: smell.

A gateway to the mind, scents are recognized more quickly than pain and remembered more permanently than sight, more precisely than sound. Differing from the other senses that travel in circuitous routes, aromas in the air are carried directly to that area of the brain responsible for emotion and memory, the limbic system. This oldest and most primitive part of the brain—developed more than 70 million years ago, before intellectual functioning arose in the cortex—was originally called the rhinencephalon or "smell brain." The limbic system is now known to control not only emotional response but, through its connections to the endocrine and autonomic nervous systems, all the primordial drives—hunger, thirst, sexuality—as well as the unconscious bodily functions necessary for survival, including respiration, circulation, and digestion.

Although awareness of an odor quickly fades or tires after exposure, nevertheless the mind is led, albeit unconsciously, by smell. Once prescribed only by high priests who alone were considered worthy of dispensing their powers, essential oils have been used throughout the ages to subtly but profoundly modulate mood and emotion. The oils may be classified into five general categories based on their overall effects on mind and body:

Relaxing
Uplifting
Harmonizing
Stimulating
Arousing

According to ancient Greek classifications still used today, some aromatic oils are relaxing, calming fears or irritability and soothing away tension. Others are uplifting to the spirits, encouraging a renewed optimism and zest for living. Certain oils are harmonizing, either relaxing or enlivening depending on need, or balancing during periods of disequilibrium. Some are mentally stimulating, sharpening concentration and clear thinking or improving memory, as well as physically energizing and invigorating. Others arouse feelings of love or passion, inspire creativity, or enhance spirituality. Most awaken sensuality by the loveliness of their scent and help promote a state of inner receptivity where, aware and connected, a moment may be more fully felt.

These essential oils—fragrance, pure and simple—may be easily enjoyed by the sensuous woman who chooses to create a still time and place for pleasure amidst the cares and distractions of daily life. For this woman, fragrance—whether sprinkled in the bath, applied as an unguent to the face, massaged on the body, worn as perfume, or wafted through the air—is part of a love affair with living, and a glorious celebration of its gifts to treasure and to share.

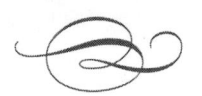

Relaxing Oils

Cedarwood

Chamomile

Clary Sage

Cypress

Frankincense

Jasmine

Lavender

Marjoram

Neroli

Rose

Sandalwood

Vetivert

Ylang Ylang

Uplifting Oils

Basil

Bergamot

Clary Sage

Clove

Geranium

Grapefruit

Jasmine

Juniper

Lemon

Orange

Patchouli

Pine

Rosemary

Harmonizing Oils

Bergamot

Cedarwood

Frankincense

Geranium

Lavender

Melissa

Rose

Stimulating Oils

Basil

Black Pepper

Clove

Grapefruit

Juniper

Lemon

Peppermint

Rosemary

Thyme

Arousing Oils

Black Pepper

Cedarwood

Clary Sage

Clove

Jasmine

Neroli

Patchouli

Pine

Rose

Sandalwood

Vetivert

Ylang Ylang

In Fragrant Water
Aromatic Baths

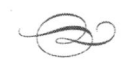

Water—the substance from which all life arose and through which all life receives sustenance—stirs ancient memories of the far distant past when humanity was still one with the sea. Used throughout time as a universal symbol of the Source, water is the wellspring of existence, the nurturing womb of life.

Submerged in the soft sanctuary of water, released from the weight of matter, cleansed and purified, the mind and the spirit may be set free to seek what the heart desires. Be it solitude or intimacy, the ethereal or the earthy, immersion in water allows for a safe refuge and a still time apart to pause, to contemplate, to explore the ordinary and the extraordinary.

A sojourn in the foreign yet familiar liquid world of water, whether the sea, a sacred river, a pure mountain stream, or a private bath, thus always contains an opportunity for the sensuous woman. Especially when fragranced with essential oils chosen not only for their beauty but for their power to evoke emotion, a mundane bath may be transformed into a magical experience where reveries float like fairies in deep waters and secret longings rise triumphantly to the light.

Several particularly inspiring aromatic baths are presented here. These bath blends are designed to encourage an exploration either inward to greater self-awareness or outward to fuller participation with another. But the final selection of the oils, like the journey itself, is a personal one—one that is both part of the process as well as part of the pleasure.

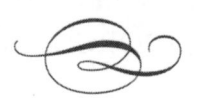

Return to the Source

To relax in a gently rocking cradle of water, to delve deeply into the center of the self and here to find the source, and finally to emerge from this contemplative space refreshed and renewed . . .

. . . sprinkle in a full bath

Vetivert, 1 drop

Frankincense, 3 drops

Orange, 2 drops

This grounding and relaxing aromatic bath promotes feelings of inner calm and centeredness while freeing the psyche to explore the hidden recesses of consciousness or the higher planes of spiritual awareness. A bath blend that inspires meditation, even revelation, the combination of vetivert, frankincense, and orange ultimately restores a zest for living now.

• • •

. . . sprinkle in a full bath

Chamomile, 2 drops

Neroli, 4 drops

A bath containing chamomile and the exquisite neroli is profoundly soothing and stabilizing. A lighter, less spiritual blend than vetivert, frankincense, and orange, this combination helps create a peaceful state of equilibrium in which the inner voice can be more clearly heard.

• • •

. . . sprinkle in a full bath

Cedarwood, 3 drops

Lavender, 3 drops

Bathing in the oil of the ancient cedar-wood tree, especially when combined with the harmonizing and healing essence of lavender, is quietly strengthening and comforting. This blend is particularly effective at encouraging integration and self-esteem through acceptance and love of the self and others.

Still Waters of Tranquility

*To let go of cares and, with the mind still,
to descend into a quiet place within, and in
this sanctuary to rest and recover . . .*

. . . sprinkle in a full bath

Lavender, 2 drops

Frankincense, 2 drops

Neroli, 2 drops

These fragrant oils clear the mind of negative or agitated thoughts as well as slow down and smooth out heightened emotions. Perhaps best suited to a nighttime bath, lavender, frankincense, and neroli instill a sense of heavenly tranquility and calm well-being.

• • •

. . . sprinkle in a full bath

Marjoram, 3 drops

Lavender, 2 drops

Geranium, 1 drop

This bath blend, like the one above, helps dispel negativity but is less cerebral and more concerned with sedating the senses. The combination of the deeply relaxing oils of marjoram and lavender with the balancing properties of geranium provide a warm, secure atmosphere in which the mind and emotions may be switched off, realigned, and replenished.

Surrender to the Pleasure

To feel at ease in the soft undulating water,
to languish in the luxurious sensations of
the moment and to be slowly awakened . . .

. . . sprinkle in a full bath

Patchouli, 1 drop

Rose, 3 drops

Bergamot, 2 drops

An exotic and erotic blend that combines the earthy powerfulness of patchouli with the feminine, unfolding seductiveness of rose, these oils help release a sensuality that is individual and uninhibited. A bath with this tantalizing blend ignites the spark of passionate love and leaves behind a lingering glow.

• • •

. . . sprinkle in a full bath

Clary Sage, 2 drops

Melissa, 2 drops

Cedarwood, 2 drops

This highly evocative combination liberates the emotions to uncover not only the sensual but the sexual, and opens the heart to the possibility of love and the joy of life it inspires.

Celebration of Desire

To lie in perfumed waters and experience the full flowering of desire, to await the mystery of another and to wish for union as the fertile sea beckons its rhythmic partner the moon . . .

. . . sprinkle in a full bath

Sandalwood, 2 drops

Ylang Ylang, 2 drops

Jasmine, 1 drop

Black Pepper, 1 drop

A bath for lovers, this seductive scent excites the imagination, arouses the senses, and builds the stamina to prolong the pleasure.

● ● ●

. . . sprinkle in a full bath

Rose, 2 drops

Jasmine, 1 drop

Sandalwood, 2 drops

Bergamot, 1 drop

A lavish, costly blend best reserved for the most heart-stopping encounters, the combination of these scents not only enhances sexual enjoyment but raises the likelihood of reproduction—the power of nature pulsating behind all temptation.

Radiant Vitality

To see the colors of life and hear the birds' song, to be centered, confident, and empowered—ready for action, revitalized...

... sprinkle in a full bath

Thyme, 2 drops

Rosemary, 2 drops

Grapefruit, 2 drops

These three stimulating and invigorating oils recharge the batteries both mentally and physically. A vibrant, energy-boosting blend, the fragrance of this combination reverberates with the optimism of a clear and sunny day.

• • •

... sprinkle in a full bath

Orange, 2 drops

Juniper, 3 drops

Black Pepper, 1 drop

A bath with orange, juniper, and black pepper cleanses and protects against the draining, energy-sapping effects of negativity so that natural vitality and exuberance can return unburdened, refocused, and committed to action.

Baths for Everyday

These aromatic baths help a woman find the best in herself—and enjoy the best in every day.

Enter Smiling

Sprinkle in a full bath.

Geranium, 2 drops

Orange, 2 drops

Bergamot, 2 drops

This light, refreshing bath blend is ideal before any social occasion where the aim is confidence and cheerfulness.

Faith in the Future

Sprinkle in a full bath.

Cedarwood, 2 drops

Cypress, 2 drops

Sandalwood, 2 drops

A bath with these mellow, soothing essences from the forest helps engender faith in the future without the need for control.

Banish the Blues

Sprinkle in a full bath.

Bergamot, 3 drops
Geranium, 2 drops
Basil, 1 drop

Bathing in these warmly uplifting aromatic oils helps rebalance even the lowest emotional states and adds a note of much-needed hope and optimism.

Evoke the Muse

Sprinkle in a full bath.

Juniper, 2 drops
Clary Sage, 2 drops
Rosemary, 2 drops

This vivid blend of elevating, inspiring oils helps free the mind of fear so that the muse may enter.

Sheer Bliss

Sprinkle in a full bath.

Rose, 2 drops
Jasmine, 2 drops
Neroli, 2 drops

A bath filled with the essence of hundreds of flowers, this precious blend evokes a sense of wonder and sheer bliss.

Guidelines for Using
Aromatic Oils in the Bath

The essential oils are pure products of nature and their effects are profound yet subtle. Less is often more, and a combination of 3–4 oils is generally sufficient when added to the bath. While the maximum number of drops for each essential oil is listed in the tables, the total number should not exceed 6–8 drops in a full bath. The oils may be dispersed directly in a full bath—a running bath unnecessarily speeds up evaporation of the fragrances—or first combined with 1 teaspoon of a base oil, such as sweet almond oil or grapeseed oil. While not soluble in water, the aromatic oils form fragrant droplets that float on the surface to lightly perfume the skin, delight the senses, and free the mind and emotions for an extraordinary bath.

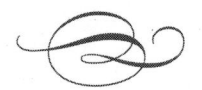

Relaxing Oils for the Bath

Aromatic Oil, Max. Drops/Full Bath

Cedarwood, 2–3

Chamomile, 2–3

Clary Sage, 2

Cypress, 4

Frankincense, 5–6

Jasmine, 3

Lavender, 5–6

Marjoram, 5–6

Neroli, 3–4

Rose, 3

Sandalwood, 5–6

Vetivert, 1–2

Ylang Ylang, 4

Uplifting Oils for the Bath

Aromatic Oil, Max. Drops/Full Bath

Basil, 2–3

Bergamot*, 2–3

Clary Sage, 2

Geranium, 3–4

Grapefruit*, 3–4

Jasmine, 3

Juniper, 4

Lemon*, 1–2

Orange*, 3

Patchouli, 1–2

Pine, 2–3

Rosemary, 3–4

Avoid using before exposure to direct sunlight

Harmonizing Oils for the Bath

Aromatic Oil, Max. Drops/Full Bath

Bergamot*, 2–3

Cedarwood, 2–3

Frankincense, 5–6

Geranium, 3–4

Lavender, 5–6

Melissa, 2–3

Rose, 3

Avoid using before exposure to direct sunlight

Stimulating Oils for the Bath

Aromatic Oil, Max. Drops/Full Bath

Basil, 2–3

Black Pepper, 2–3

Grapefruit*, 3–4

Juniper, 4

Lemon*, 1–2

Peppermint, 1–2

Rosemary, 3–4

Thyme, 3

Avoid using before exposure to direct sunlight

Arousing Oils for the Bath

Aromatic Oil, Max. Drops/Full Bath

Black Pepper, 2–3

Cedarwood, 2–3

Clary Sage, 2

Jasmine, 3

Neroli, 3–4

Patchouli, 1–2

Pine, 2–3

Rose, 3

Sandalwood, 5–6

Vetivert, 1–2

Ylang Ylang, 3–4

Luminous and Lovely
Fragrant Oils for the Face

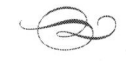

As the blossom identifies the plant, so the face is the embodiment of the woman. The focal point for expression and communication, the face reflects the true nature, the character, the life story, and the deepest desires of the woman behind it. For most, the intimacy of what the face reveals causes an almost instinctive need to hide the more painful traces of life's legacy. Yet what attracts in a face, as in a blossom, is not its perfection but its mystery, and the light of goodness, humor, daring, and intelligence that radiates from the person like the fragrance from a flower. How captivating is the woman who freely, unselfconsciously, shows her face to the world!

Fragrant oils, which act holistically on all levels of being—body, mind, and spirit—have been used in facial unguents since antiquity. Once prescribed with great care and ceremony, an aromatic oil for the face was chosen not only for its action on the skin but also for its effects on the mind and emotions. The oils may be used in the same way today to improve the health of the skin and the overall well-being of the woman, so that the light of individual loveliness may more clearly shine through.

Because of their small and compatible molecular structure, the essential oils penetrate through the outer layer of the skin to help promote normal, balanced functioning. As unique as their scent, each essential oil has its own particular properties that may be beneficial to the skin, whether regenerative, restorative, rebalancing, or rejuvenating. Especially when combined with a nourishing base oil, an aromatic formulation used consistently on the face can have effects as stunning as its fragrance.

Facial unguents for women with normal, dry, oily, and mature skin are presented here. Although the selection of oils obviously depends on their ability to nurture, nourish, clean, and tone the skin, the fragrance of each blend is also designed to enhance the woman's joyful participation in the creative process of change — of evolving over time, like the blossom, from expectant bud to full flower and beyond.

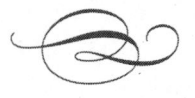

Nurturing Normal Skin

To nurture a well-balanced skin, neither dry nor oily, dehydrated nor moist, for a face clearly reflecting the light and loveliness, the health and vitality of the woman who cares for it . . .

. . . *combine*

Geranium, 1 drop
Lavender, 2 drops
Sweet almond oil or
unperfumed moisturizer,
1 tablespoon

The naturally balancing oil of geranium and the exceptionally regenerative properties of lavender make this facial unguent a superb choice for women with the gift, either natural or acquired, of great-looking skin. With a fragrance as tranquil as a summer's stroll through a swaying field of lavender, this soothing yet uplifting blend helps induce a peaceful sense of integration, the hallmark of a healthy woman.

Nourishing Dry Skin

*To nourish and enrich dry skin for a face
soft to the touch, even in texture and color,
eased of restraint, and freely expressing the
woman's unique beauty and multifaceted
femininity...*

... combine

Neroli, 2 drops

Chamomile, 1 drop

Sweet almond oil or

unperfumed moisturizer,

1 tablespoon

One of the most costly and luxurious of
oils, neroli is also one of the most nourishing. Particularly when combined with
healing chamomile, this blend excels at
restoring natural lubrication to dry skin.
In addition, the delicate fragrance of
orange blossoms and sunny chamomile
helps promote a state of inner calm
where, with tenderness and patience, the
character of the woman so finely etched
in her face may be gracefully accepted.

Clearing Oily Skin

To clear congested, oily skin for a face smooth and unblemished, bright and lustrous, radiating the quiet confidence of a woman unmasked and willing to reveal . . .

. . . *combine*

Sandalwood, 2 drops

Juniper, 1 drop

Sweet almond oil or

unperfumed moisturizer,

1 tablespoon

The soothing yet gently astringent sandalwood and the detoxifying juniper create an ideal blend for healing often fussed-over oily skin. The empowering fragrance of this facial unguent similarly helps to clear away negativity and inhibitions and increase the woman's confidence to shine both inwardly and outwardly.

Toning Mature Skin

*To tone and rejuvenate mature skin, for a
firmer, more elastic, less lined face, glowing
with the secrets and surprises of a woman
still sensuous and ready to smile . . .*

. . . combine

Frankincense, 2 drops

Rose, 1 drop

Sweet almond oil or

unperfumed moisturizer,

1 tablespoon

Proven on pharaohs to preserve the skin,
frankincense is the aromatic oil par excellence for toning mature skin. Worthy of
Queen Cleopatra, this exquisite blend
adds a velvety plumpness to the skin
while its sublimely feminine fragrance
evokes not only love for others but for the
special beauty of a well-lived face.

Uplifting Facial Toners

These fragrant facial toners for dry and oily skin help refresh the face and revive the spirits.

Lubricating Rosewater Toner

Combine and shake well before each use.

Rose, 1 drop

Chamomile, 1 drop

Rosewater, 3 tablespoons

Like the morning dew on a rose petal, this aromatic toner protects dry skin and leaves the face feeling silky smooth, and the woman feeling wonderful.

Liberating Orange Flower Water Toner

Combine and shake well before each use.

Sandalwood, 1 drop

Lavender, 1 drop

Orange flower water, 3 tablespoons

This light floral water helps free the skin of blemishes and return a healthy sheen and luster to the woman's lovely face.

Guidelines for Using
Aromatic Oils on the Face

Essential oils must always be diluted in a base oil, such as sweet almond oil or commercial unperfumed moisturizers. If the skin is especially dry, a few drops of avocado oil may be incorporated to enrich the blend; if excessively oily, the more astringent grapeseed oil may be used. Facial unguents penetrate best if applied to a slightly damp face and neck using gentle upward strokes, with care taken not to drag or pull the skin, especially around the eyes.

Because of the delicacy of the skin on the face, essential oils are used more sparingly than on other areas of the body. The maximum number of drops for each essential oil is listed in the tables, but the total number should not exceed 3 drops per 1 tablespoon of base oil. This provides roughly two weeks' supply of unguent for the face and neck that, like all aromatic formulations, stay fresh and fragrant longest if stored in dark glass containers away from heat and light.

Consistent use of the essential oil is crucial: outward signs of improvement usually take at least thirty days as the plump new skin cells travel upward from the basal layer, where they are produced, to the outer epidermis. With attention and patience, however, these precious essences quietly work their wonders on the skin so that the essence of the woman—her inner light and loveliness—may be reflected in her face.

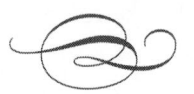

Aromatic Oils for Normal Skin

Aromatic Oil, Max. Drops/1 Tbsp. Base Oil

Frankincense, 3

Geranium, 2

Lavender, 3

Neroli, 2

Rose, 2

Rosemary, 1

Ylang Ylang, 2

Aromatic Oils for Dry Skin

Aromatic Oil, Max. Drops/1 Tbsp. Base Oil

Chamomile, 2

Clary Sage, 1

Frankincense, 3

Geranium, 2

Jasmine, 2

Lavender, 3

Neroli, 2

Rose, 2

Sandalwood, 3

Ylang Ylang, 2

Aromatic Oils for Oily Skin

Aromatic Oil, Max. Drops/1 Tbsp. Base Oil

Clary Sage, 1

Cypress, 2

Frankincense, 3

Geranium, 2

Juniper, 1

Lavender, 3

Neroli, 2

Patchouli, 1

Rose, 2

Rosemary, 1

Sandalwood, 3

Ylang Ylang, 2

Aromatic Oils for Mature Skin

Aromatic Oil, Max. Drops/1 Tbsp. Base Oil

Clary Sage, 1

Cypress, 2

Frankincense, 3

Geranium, 2

Lavender, 3

Neroli, 2

Patchouli, 1

Rose, 2

Rosemary, 1

Sandalwood, 3

Vetivert, 1

Ylang Ylang, 2

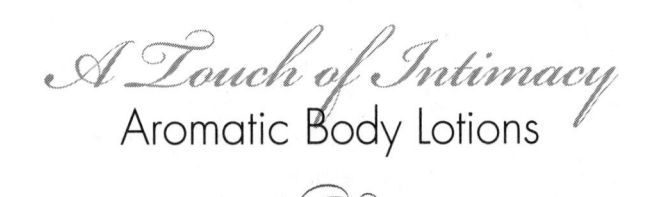

A Touch of Intimacy
Aromatic Body Lotions

Like an explorer, solitary and at sea, the self encased in the physical body longs to reach out and discover another. To cross the barriers and enter the uncharted waters of the mysterious other, this daring adventure often begins with only a touch. An instant of connection, touch conveys not only the temperature, texture, pressure, and vibration of flesh, but also the mind, emotions, and spirit of the traveler in these realms.

The first sense of the embryo, touch is the elemental force that bonds. In a language more ancient, more powerful, more accurate than words, touch communicates the fullness and the reality of the self to another so that forever after there is recognition. Touch is the language of intimacy, of knowing and being known—a language fluent to all, understood by all, yet all too frequently forgotten or left unspoken.

Although often relegated to the purely sexual or the merely functional, touch with intention—touch that relays the messages of the person—carries within it the potential not only for intimacy but also for love. A gentle reassuring touch, a light hopeful touch—a touch that transfers feelings, a touch that *feels*—can overcome the obstacles of physical separateness and unite, however briefly, two souls who are no longer alone.

To touch the body without criticism but with affection and appreciation, to be in touch with the needs of the body and with kindness respond to those needs, this *self-centeredness* is a crucial prerequisite not only for health but for healthy interaction with another.

Essential oils for the body combine the intimacy of touch with the powerfully evocative effects of fragrance to create a doubly enticing experience. Whether stimulating or soothing, uplifting, inspiring, empowering or exciting, the aromatic blends presented here help encourage a touch that is touching to the body and the spirit—a touch that touches the heart of another.

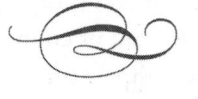

Being in Touch

To feel connected to the physical body and responsive to its needs for energy, rest, and regeneration, apply with a respectful, grateful touch . . .

A New Day
. . . combine

Rosemary, 2 drops

Juniper, 2 drops

Lemon, 2 drops

Sweet almond oil or

unperfumed body lotion, 1 tablespoon

This crisp, clean, fresh scent awakens the body and mind for an invigorating start to the day, especially if challenging, draining, or even unpleasant situations lie ahead.

Strength and Stamina
. . . combine

Black pepper, 1 drop

Rosemary, 4 drops

Sweet almond oil or

unperfumed body lotion, 1 tablespoon

Before arduous physical activity—a sports event, long jog, or day outdoors—a body rub with this super-energizing blend strengthens the body and increases stamina.

Calm and Centered

... combine

Vetivert, 2 drops
Neroli, 4 drops
Sweet almond oil or
unperfumed body lotion, 1 tablespoon

If anxious or overwhelmed, the hauntingly beautiful and harmonizing blend of vetivert and neroli helps instill an inner calm, a sense of centeredness, and a renewed tranquility.

Soothing Stress and Strain

... combine

Lavender, 3 drops
Marjoram, 3 drops
Sweet almond oil or
unperfumed body lotion, 1 tablespoon

This warm and deeply soothing body oil eases tight muscles and relaxes a tense mind so that the stresses and strains of the day may be put in perspective and set aside.

Evening of Dancing
...combine

Geranium, 2 drops

Orange, 2 drops

Rosemary, 2 drops

Sweet almond oil or

unperfumed body lotion, 1 tablespoon

A cheerful and reviving blend, the aromatic combination of geranium, orange, and rosemary lifts the mood in readiness for laughter and an evening of dancing.

A Good Night
...combine

Frankincense, 3 drops

Lavender, 3 drops

Sweet almond oil or

unperfumed body lotion, 1 tablespoon

The oils of frankincense and lavender promote a restful sleep that gives the body time to recuperate and frees the mind to dream.

Touching the Spirit

To reach down into the elemental spheres of being and there to find the seeds of joy and harmony, apply with a loving touch . . .

Enjoy the Moment

. . . combine

Orange, 3 drops

Cedarwood, 3 drops

Sweet almond oil or

unperfumed body lotion, 1 tablespoon

While joy is sometimes experienced as a surprise, most often it arrives when asked for and recognized in the beauty of the moment. A relaxing yet enlivening blend, these oils encourage a firm grounding in the present and an unreserved vitality for living.

Gentle Boost

. . . combine

Grapefruit, 3 drops

Geranium, 3 drops

Sweet almond oil or

unperfumed body lotion, 1 tablespoon

When feeling low, the combination of grapefruit and geranium helps to equalize the ebb and flow of emotions with its sunny and uplifting scent.

Essence of Harmony
... combine

Frankincense, 2 drops
Sandalwood, 3 drops
Geranium, 1 drop
Sweet almond oil or
unperfumed body lotion, 1 tablespoon

The ancient oils of frankincense and sandalwood, used for millennia to quiet the mind and emotions for contemplation, when combined with the balancing effects of geranium create a blend that inspires peacefulness and harmony.

Simply Oneself
... combine

Bergamot, 3 drops
Jasmine, 2 drops
Sweet almond oil or
unperfumed body lotion, 1 tablespoon

A light, exquisite fragrance, this aromatic blend helps restore positive feelings of clarity and optimism, and the confidence to simply be oneself.

Touching Another

To communicate in a language beyond words and explore with exuberance the unknown territory of another, apply with a trusting, instinctual touch . . .

Come Hither
. . . combine

Orange, 3 drops

Neroli, 3 drops

Sweet almond oil or

unperfumed body lotion, 1 tablespoon

The oils from the fruit and flower of the orange tree have an irresistibly seductive scent that is fully feminine and alluring.

The Mood for Love
. . . combine

Rose, 3 drops

Sandalwood, 3 drops

Sweet almond oil or

unperfumed body lotion, 1 tablespoon

These two precious aphrodisiacs cleanse the mind of distracting thoughts, and set a mood for sensuous pleasure and slow, romantic love.

Romantic Encounters

. . . combine

Ylang Ylang, 2 drops
Jasmine, 2 drops
Bergamot, 2 drops
Sweet almond oil or
unperfumed body lotion, 1 tablespoon

A super-sexy scent for lovers who crave communion as well as release, this aromatic blend is renowned for facilitating both union and reunion after times of separation or sadness.

Lovely to Touch

These fragrant body lotions help keep the body looking lovely—and lovely to touch.

A Beautiful Back

Form a paste and rub into a clean, damp back using gentle circular movements, then rinse off.

Lavender, 2 drops

Lemon, 1 drop

Sweet almond oil, 1 teaspoon

Oatmeal, 1 tablespoon

Ground almonds, 1 tablespoon

For a tinglingly clean back that is beautiful and blemish-free, apply this aromatic blend once or twice weekly.

Caressable Breasts

Gently massage the breasts in outward circular movements toward the underarms.

Ylang Ylang, 1 drop

Sweet almond oil, 1 teaspoon

According to Eastern folklore, a massage with ylang ylang helps keep the breasts firm and youthful.

Healing Hands
Combine.

Rose, 1 drop

Jojoba, 1 teaspoon

This rich, fragrant blend is deeply moisturizing for soft, gentle hands.

Pretty Feet
Combine.

Lavender, 2 drops

Sweet almond oil, 1 teaspoon

A foot massage with lavender not only soothes tired, aching feet but keeps them soft and smooth for barefoot summer days.

Guidelines for Using
Aromatic Oils on the Body

Sweet almond oil, which is extremely nourishing, or non-greasy commercial unperfumed body lotion are suggested as base oils for the body. If a more moisturizing blend is required for particularly dry skin, the blend may be enriched by adding ½ teaspoon of either avocado oil or jojoba to 1 tablespoon of base oil. The maximum number of drops for each essential oil is listed in the tables, but the total number should not exceed 6 drops per tablespoon of base oil. If more convenient, 1 tablespoon is equivalent to an approximate handful of base oil, and the drops of aromatic oil may be blended directly in the palm of the hand before each use.

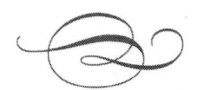

Relaxing Oils for the Body

Aromatic Oil, Max. Drops/1 Tbsp. Base Oil

Cedarwood, 3

Chamomile, 3

Clary Sage, 3

Cypress, 4

Frankincense, 6

Jasmine, 3

Lavender, 6

Marjoram, 6

Neroli, 3–4

Rose, 3

Sandalwood, 6

Vetivert, 2

Ylang Ylang, 4

Uplifting Oils for the Body

Aromatic Oil, Max. Drops/1 Tbsp. Base Oil

Basil, 3

Bergamot*, 3

Clary Sage, 3

Geranium, 3

Grapefruit*, 3

Jasmine, 3

Juniper, 4

Lemon*, 2

Orange*, 3

Patchouli, 2

Pine, 3

Rosemary, 3–4

Avoid using before exposure to direct sunlight

Harmonizing Oils for the Body

Aromatic Oil, Max. Drops/1 Tbsp. Base Oil

Bergamot*, 3

Cedarwood, 3

Frankincense, 6

Geranium, 3

Lavender, 6

Melissa, 3

Rose, 3

Avoid using before exposure to direct sunlight

Stimulating Oils for the Body

Aromatic Oil, Max. Drops/1 Tbsp. Base Oil

Basil, 3

Black Pepper, 3

Grapefruit*, 3

Juniper, 4

Lemon*, 2

Peppermint, 2

Rosemary, 3–4

Thyme, 3

Avoid using before exposure to direct sunlight

Arousing Oils for the Body

Aromatic Oil, Max. Drops/1 Tbsp. Base Oil

Black Pepper, 3

Cedarwood, 3

Clary Sage, 3

Jasmine, 3

Neroli, 3–4

Patchouli, 2

Pine, 3

Rose, 3

Sandalwood, 6

Vetivert, 2

Ylang Ylang, 4

Behind the Fragrant Veil
Perfumes

From the Greek *pherein*, "to carry," and *horman*, "to excite," the human scent of pheromones is arousing on a primal physical plane. Deeply alluring, like the flower's fragrance to the bee, the individual scent of female essence signals that which is essential for survival: her readiness or receptivity to mate. Sweeter during ovulation, magnetic during stimulation, pheromones are perhaps nature's most provocative perfume.

Physically compelling, yet limited in scope — describing the unconscious and the instinctual but omitting the psyche and the soul — the scent of pheromones has throughout the ages been enhanced by the fragrant oils of aromatic plants. These powerfully evocative oils, when intermingled with the natural body scent, create an aura of aroma that silently conveys the spirit of the woman.

Like a veil of fragrance, the perfumes of aromatic oils tantalize and seduce by hinting at the hidden, mysterious woman behind the veil. Transmuting the physical dimension of scent into the ether of illusion, perfumes paint in fragrance a portrait of the woman that both highlights an aspect of herself and inspires, through scent alone, the imagination of another.

Several suggestions for perfumes composed of the pure fragrance of essential oils are presented here. These perfume blends are formulated to express various archetypes of the female psyche passed through in a lifetime or a day, inherent if not evident in all women. They excite, like the woman herself, moods and emotions of playfulness, passion, and awe. Yet, however captivating in their fragrant illusion, these beautiful perfumes represent only a few generalized conceptions of a woman, and not a specific self-image. To create this—a self-portrait in perfume—is an artistic endeavor that may be undertaken by any woman who desires to communicate, through the abstraction of scent, a facet of her femininity, her complexity, and her formidable capacity to love.

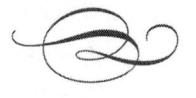

Mischief

To retrieve the Playful Maiden, vibrant and vivacious, charming others with her spontaneity, innocently wielding her power like a wand, unaffected and unafraid, fearlessly loving, mischievous . . .

. . . combine

Bergamot, 8 drops

Lemon, 6 drops

Rosemary, 4 drops

Lavender, 4 drops

Neroli, 3 drops

Jojoba, 1 tablespoon

This lightly romantic perfume has a lively, fresh fragrance that evokes a carefree playfulness, like a romp through a field of red poppies.

• • •

. . . combine

Orange, 8 drops

Cypress, 5 drops

Juniper, 5 drops

Sandalwood, 7 drops

Jojoba, 1 tablespoon

A cheerful and uplifting perfume with a distinctly woody fragrance, the combination of these aromatic oils conjures up an enchanted forest immune to time where creative muses, sensual nymphs, and spirit gods are free to frolic.

Temptation

*To summon Aphrodite, supremely sensual
and seductive, shimmering with irresistible
femininity, magnetically alluring — the
source of temptation, the goddess of love . . .*

. . . combine

Rose, 4 drops

Jasmine, 4 drops

Neroli, 4 drops

Jojoba, 1 tablespoon

Exquisitely floral and enticing, a perfume of rose, jasmine, and neroli conveys a characteristically feminine sensuality that balances generosity with
receptivity and passion with love.

• • •

. . . combine

Ylang Ylang, 8 drops

Bergamot, 8 drops

Rose, 4 drops

Jojoba, 1 tablespoon

Ylang ylang, an exotic floral fragrance of
the South Seas, stimulates a desire that
longs for release. As the fire of the male
is said to heat the water of the female, so
this intoxicating perfume both quickens
and quenches the flame.

Abandon

To unleash the Wild Woman, untamed and uninhibited, overflowing with pure sexual energy, exuberant and free, alive with abandon . . .

. . . combine

Orange, 8 drops

Patchouli, 4 drops

Frankincense, 6 drops

Ylang Ylang, 4 drops

Jojoba, 1 tablespoon

Earthy and mysterious, the instinctual, unconventional, and powerfully provocative quality of this perfume is deeply fascinating and disturbing.

• • •

. . . combine

Bergamot, 8 drops

Black Pepper, 4 drops

Jasmine, 4 drops

Sandalwood, 7 drops

Jojoba, 1 tablespoon

Less earthy and physical but equally intense, the complex combination of citrus and spice, flower and wood produces a fragrance of pervasive sexuality that is freely expressive and full of joy.

Esteem

To release the Powerful Woman, crusader and champion, confident, courageous, with a will transformed to action and a zeal for living—energetic, assertive, and highly esteemed . . .

. . . combine

Orange, 8 drops

Grapefruit, 6 drops

Black Pepper, 4 drops

Cedarwood, 6 drops

Jojoba, 1 tablespoon

An invigorating perfume with a zesty, spicy, somewhat masculine character, this uplifting blend stimulates, strengthens, and empowers, especially if the challenge is creative or intellectual.

• • •

. . . combine

Lemon, 7 drops

Black Pepper, 3 drops

Juniper, 5 drops

Rosemary, 5 drops

Jojoba, 1 tablespoon

A perfume with a clear, refreshing fragrance reminiscent of the great outdoors, the combination of these oils helps to cleanse the mind of negativity, trigger the will, and encourage courageous action. A powerful perfume for a powerful woman!

Devotion

*To celebrate the Great Goddess Earth,
warm and womanly, ripe with life and res-
onating love, abundantly generous yet con-
tinually plentiful, the object of devotion . . .*

. . . combine

Lemon, 7 drops

Geranium, 4 drops

Lavender, 6 drops

Frankincense, 6 drops

Jojoba, 1 tablespoon

This lovely perfume has a comforting
floral scent with a slightly earthy undertone that stabilizes the natural rhythms
of the emotions, soothes the psyche, and
inspires quiet gratitude.

• • •

. . . combine

Rose, 2 drops

Rosewater, 1 tablespoon

Rose—the Queen of Flowers, the most
feminine of fragrances, and the embodiment of perfume—is the essence of the
Earth Mother, creator and nurturer,
rooted to the soil, in harmony with the
stars.

Serenity

*To call upon the Wise Woman, enlightened
and evolving, inspiring love for life and joy
in the moment, the healer sought after and
adored, radiant and serene . . .*

. . . combine

Orange, 8 drops

Bergamot, 8 drops

Rose, 4 drops

Frankincense, 5 drops

Jojoba, 1 tablespoon

With a lingering aura of the mystical and
the sublime, this mysterious perfume
aids the journey inward through contemplation and the journey outward through
love.

•   •   •

. . . combine

Bergamot, 8 drops

Melissa, 5 drops

Lavender, 7 drops

Neroli, 5 drops

Jojoba, 1 tablespoon

The joyful scent of this perfume encourages a sense of peaceful integration and
helps light the path to love and the
serenity it bestows.

Perfumed Hair —
A Fragrant Seduction

The hair, framing the face like the feathers of a peacock, displays a sexuality that intends to seduce. Covered over in cultures where female sexuality is feared or exalted in those where it is considered the foundation of female power, the hair expresses much about the woman and her relationship to the instinctive, utterly female aspects of herself.

Since antiquity, and perhaps always, the hair has been dyed, colored, curled, braided, waxed, powdered, oiled, and adorned—with beads, jewels, ribbons, combs, or flowers—as part of a ritual of temptation no less fantastic than the most brilliant of plumages. Aromatic oils to subtly perfume the hair have been used for millennia to increase sensual pleasure, whether modulating mood as fingers moving through the hair waft up aroma, or enhancing the delight of burying the face in another's hair. The following fragrant rinses perfume the hair for every day, or for those splendid encounters with another when the moment of seduction and release may be made more lovely, more joyous through scent.

The following essential oils are best mixed in a bowl of warm water and used as a final rinse on freshly shampooed hair. Contact with the eyes should be avoided.

A Sprinkling of Magic
Sprinkle in a bowl of warm water.

Rosemary, 6 drops

Like the kiss of a fairy prince, this reviving and empowering scent stimulates awakening.

A Sprinkling of Mystery
Sprinkle in a bowl of warm water.

Frankincense, 6 drops

The warm, inspiring fragrance of frankincense hints at the hidden and the mysterious, like an oasis deep in its desert habitat.

A Sprinkling of Fantasy

Sprinkle in a bowl of warm water.

Sandalwood, 6 drops

A revered aphrodisiac in the East, sandalwood stimulates inclination and expands the imagination for an added sensual dimension.

A Sprinkling of Passion

Sprinkle in a bowl of warm water.

Ylang Ylang, 4 drops

Jasmine, 2 drops

Two of the most exotic and provocative aromatic oils, the fragrance of ylang ylang and jasmine captures the irresistibility of night-scented blossoms and the intensity of passionate love.

A Sprinkling of Love

Sprinkle in a bowl of warm water.

Rose, 3 drops

Sandalwood, 3 drops

A truly sublime fragrance that is both feminine and masculine, this is a deeply magnetic blend for lovers in unison.

Guidelines for Using
Aromatic Oils as Perfumes

Aromatic oils have varying rates of evaporation, classified as top, middle, and base notes. The lightest, most volatile oils, or top notes, are noticed first in a perfume blend but disappear most quickly, while heavier base notes linger the longest and are the slowest to evaporate. Between these, the middle notes typically comprise the fragrant heart of the blend. A harmonious perfume that creates an illusion of depth and complexity generally results from an interplay of top, middle, and base notes, but the overall effect of the blend is obviously far more crucial than its composition by note.

Until the nineteenth century, all perfumes were composed entirely of aromatic oils. Today, because of cost, even the finest are composed predominantly of synthetic fragrances. The more expensive a perfume, the more pure fragrance it contains.

When preparing a perfume of fragrant oils, the maximum number of drops for each essential oil is listed in the tables. As a general rule, however, no more than 20–25 drops of oils should be used for every 1 tablespoon of jojoba.

The quantity of essential oils in these blends is quite high and more jojoba may be added if the scent is too strong. The perfumes can be reapplied frequently throughout the day (or night) as their fragrance, while purer, is also more fleeting than synthetically fixed commercial perfumes.

All citrus oils—especially bergamot—cause photosensitivity, and on a day full of sunshine it is wise to be cautious and restrict perfumes containing these oils to areas not exposed to the sun.

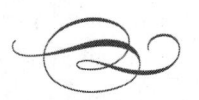

Blended in Harmony:
Classification of Aromatic Oils

Top Notes
Basil, Bergamot, Grapefruit,
Lemon, Orange

Middle Notes
Black Pepper, Chamomile, Clary Sage,
Cypress, Geranium, Juniper, Lavender,
Marjoram, Melissa, Peppermint,
Pine, Rosemary, Thyme

Base Notes
Cedarwood, Clove*, Frankincense,
Jasmine, Neroli, Patchouli, Rose,
Sandalwood, Vetivert, Ylang Ylang

Use as an air fragrancer only

Fragrance Categories

Citrus
Bergamot, Grapefruit, Lemon,
Melissa, Orange

Floral
Geranium, Jasmine, Lavender,
Neroli, Rose, Ylang Ylang

Herbal
Basil, Chamomile, Clary Sage,
Marjoram, Rosemary, Thyme

Menthol
Peppermint

Musky
Frankincense, Patchouli, Vetivert

Spicy
Black Pepper, Clove*

Woodland
Cedarwood, Cypress, Juniper,
Pine, Sandalwood

Use as an air fragrancer only

Relaxing Scents

Aromatic Oil, Max. Drops/1 Tbsp. Jojoba

Cedarwood, 6

Chamomile, 2

Clary Sage, 6

Cypress, 4–5

Frankincense, 6

Jasmine, 3–4

Lavender, 7

Marjoram, 3

Neroli, 4–5

Rose, 3–4

Sandalwood, 7

Vetivert, 4

Ylang Ylang, 8

Uplifting Scents

Aromatic Oil, Max. Drops/1 Tbsp. Jojoba

Basil, 2

Bergamot*, 8

Clary Sage, 6

Geranium, 4

Grapefruit*, 6

Jasmine, 3–4

Juniper, 5

Lemon*, 7

Orange*, 8

Patchouli, 4

Pine, 5

Rosemary, 5

Avoid using before exposure to direct sunlight

Harmonizing Scents

Aromatic Oil, Max. Drops/1 Tbsp. Jojoba

Bergamot*, 8

Cedarwood, 6

Frankincense, 6

Geranium, 4

Lavender, 7

Melissa, 5

Rose, 3–4

Avoid using before exposure to direct sunlight

Stimulating Scents

Aromatic Oil, Max. Drops/1 Tbsp. Jojoba

Basil, 2

Black Pepper, 3–4

Grapefruit*, 6

Juniper, 5

Lemon*, 7

Peppermint, 2

Rosemary, 5

Thyme, 2–3

Avoid using before exposure to direct sunlight

Arousing Scents

Aromatic Oil, Max. Drops/1 Tbsp. Jojoba

Black Pepper, 3–4

Cedarwood, 6

Clary Sage, 6

Jasmine, 3–4

Neroli, 4–5

Patchouli, 4

Pine, 5

Rose, 3–4

Sandalwood, 7

Vetivert, 4

Ylang Ylang, 8

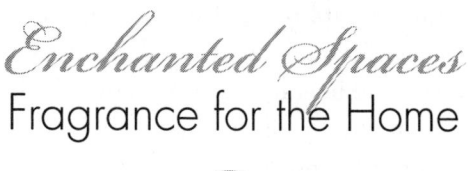

Enchanted Spaces
Fragrance for the Home

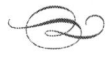

A room contains the energy of those who dwell within its walls and perhaps the remnants of those who once inhabited the space. This energy—born of human emotion, nurtured on human experience—is instantly recognizable and profoundly affecting as it flows effortlessly in an endless loop between the space and the souls who shelter there. Like a spirit in the atmosphere, the energy of a room may push away, closing its doors to ease and pleasure, or throw wide the gates, inviting expansion and joyful participation in the everyday scenarios of living.

For the woman sensitive to the forces that surround her, the energy in a room sets the stage on which the cherished daily dramas of existence are enacted. In this capacity as background for the day, influencing perspective and reaction to events, the energy in a room is regarded attentively and altered appropriately through the subtle direction of the sensuous woman. Using fragrance in the air to modulate the scene, the woman may cast out the negative, call forth the positive, and create through the powers of scent a space that is conducive to her needs, a room redolent with possibilities—an enchanted space in which to be.

Several suggestions for welcoming and evocative air fragrances are presented here to dramatically enhance the ambience of a room. These essences in the air are formulated to foster those moments at home when there is conviviality, relaxation, laughter—when love is felt in every room. Innumerable other fragrant oils may, however, be sent into the air to aromatically enthrall, transform, and liberate a space, so that the beauty inherent in the ordinary acts of living may be more intimately known.

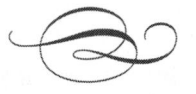

Living Room

To create a space for stillness or sociability,
full of light and free of unwanted emotions,
a room that welcomes ease and enjoyment,
conviviality and conversation . . .

Light the Candles
. . . vaporize in an oil burner

Frankincense, 2 drops

Orange, 4 drops

Sandalwood, 2 drops

This mysterious fragrance in the air sets a mood of heightened receptivity in which the preciousness of an evening — ephemeral as candlelight — may be held always in the heart.

Being with Beethoven
. . . vaporize in an oil burner

Bergamot, 3 drops

Frankincense, 3 drops

Neroli, 2 drops

The essence of contentment, this tranquil fragrance envelops a room with stillness so that the listener may merge with the music, the reader enter the story, and the dreamer become one with the dream.

Among Friends

. . . vaporize in an oil burner

Bergamot, 3 drops

Geranium, 2 drops

Lavender, 3 drops

The lively, lovely fragrance of this blend inspires an evening of harmony and conviviality where conversations flow and good-natured fellowship pervades the atmosphere.

Mysterious Stranger

. . . vaporize in an oil burner

Cedarwood, 3 drops

Lavender, 3 drops

Neroli, 2 drops

From a starting point of grounded self-awareness, the thrilling adventure of discovering another may get safely underway. This blend combines the slightly masculine scent of cedarwood with the ultrafeminine neroli to create a subtly encouraging atmosphere in which the journey to revelation and connection may slowly, and with tantalizing care, proceed.

Spontaneous Combustion

. . . vaporize in an oil burner

Black Pepper, 2 drops

Lemon, 4 drops

Ylang Ylang, 2 drops

A reliable love potion from the East, this stimulating blend conjures up the wild abandon of lush tropical nights. When sent into the atmosphere, the sensuously stirring fragrance of these oils provokes those moments of passionate spontaneity when love erupts in unexpected places.

Dining Room

To enhance a space for celebrations, sparkling with vivacity or quiet with gratitude, a room released from the concerns of the day where friends and lovers may come to share the pleasures of a meal . . .

Feast and Festivities

. . . vaporize in an oil burner

Orange, 4 drops

Geranium, 2 drops

Rosemary, 2 drops

This enlivening, uplifting fragrance in the air fills a room with high-spirited festivity conducive to laughter, generosity, and after-dinner dancing.

Saying Grace

... vaporize in an oil burner

Bergamot, 2 drops

Lemon, 2 drops

Orange, 2 drops

Sandalwood, 2 drops

The fragrance of this blend, with its familiar citrus scent and just a touch of the exotic sandalwood, helps transform a routine meal into a quiet celebration where, relaxed and unrushed, the sweet pleasures of the day may be peacefully savored.

Dinner Date

... vaporize in an oil burner

Black Pepper, 2 drops

Grapefruit, 2 drops

Jasmine, 2 drops

When dinner is a prelude to romance, the sultry fragrance of this blend captivates all suitors and stimulates flirtation—more tempting than any meal.

Study

To empower a space for concentration, clarity, and mental focus, a room for learning, creativity, and imaginative play . . .

In Focus

. . . vaporize in an oil burner

Rosemary, 2 drops

Pine, 2 drops

Lemon, 4 drops

These three stimulating fragrances not only heighten mental power but also increase the enthusiasm and determination to overcome obstacles and meet the challenges of the day.

Free to Flow

. . . vaporize in an oil burner

Lemon, 2 drops

Juniper, 2 drops

Frankincense, 2 drops

Black Pepper, 2 drops

The fragrance of lemon builds confidence, while juniper rids the mind of fear of failure. In this calmly receptive state, frankincense inspires creative thought that black pepper helps transform to art by increasing mental and physical endurance.

Dream Lover

. . . vaporize in an oil burner

Bergamot, 4 drops

Clary Sage, 2 drops

Rose, 2 drops

To release fantasies and daydreams of great delight, this blend of beautifully enticing fragrances in the air awakens desire and sets loose thoughts of passion in the most erogenous of zones.

Bedroom

To enlarge a space for wider explorations and intimate discoveries, a room where it is safe to rest, to grow, to feel the pleasure and the untamed bliss of being . . .

Finding Stillness

. . . vaporize in an oil burner

Lavender, 3 drops

Marjoram, 3 drops

These essences floating in the air form an invisible barrier to the world, creating that most precious time in which serenity may be found in stillness.

The Way Ahead

. . . vaporize in an oil burner

Bergamot, 2 drops

Cypress, 2 drops

Juniper, 2 drops

Neroli, 2 drops

In the privacy of a bedroom these comforting fragrances in the air soothe away internal turmoil and soften pain while gently lightening the atmosphere with a glowing vision of hope and faith, so simple, so elusive.

Love in the Clouds

. . . vaporize in an oil burner

Bergamot, 2 drops

Jasmine, 2 drops

Rose, 2 drops

Ylang Ylang, 2 drops

An intoxicating combination for lovers who wish to lose themselves and walk together in the clouds, this almost overwhelming fragrance of sexual yearning lingers like memories of love.

The Wonder of the Day

. . . vaporize in an oil burner

Chamomile, 1 drop

Lavender, 2 drops

Sandalwood, 3 drops

Before entering the world of dreams, these essences in the air remind the woman of those perfect moments of pure union when life filled her heart — when she and the cosmos were one.

Seasonal Scents

These fragrant blends in the air celebrate the full circle, from the newness of spring to the slumber of winter and regeneration again.

Spring

Vaporize in an oil burner.

Melissa, 3 drops

Clary Sage, 2 drops

Bergamot, 3 drops

A fragrance lightly tinged with green, this blend sparkles with the freshness of beginnings and the new growth of spring.

Summer

Vaporize in an oil burner.

Grapefruit, 4 drops

Lavender, 3 drops

Reminiscent of sun-drenched fields and shaded lawns, of long evenings when life feels wonderful, grapefruit and lavender evoke the lush essence of summer.

Fall

Vaporize in an oil burner.

Pine, 3 drops
Cedarwood, 3 drops

The combination of these deep, woody scents imbues the room with warm well-being and the quiet confidence that nature's long slumber will be safely endured.

Winter

Vaporize in an oil burner.

Orange, 4 drops
Clove, 2 drops

A delicious scent for winter festivals, orange and clove have an uplifting, enlivening scent that whispers *spring*.

Guidelines for Using
Aromatic Oils in the Air

Many techniques exist to fragrance a
room, from a bowl of boiling water that
exudes the scent as it cools to light bulb
rings and mists or sprays. A candle-heat-
ed or electrical oil burner, available
wherever essential oils are sold, is, however, the simplest and most long-lasting
way to transform a room into an
enchanted space. The maximum number
of drops for each essential oil is listed in
the tables, but generally a combination
of 3–4 oils in a total of 8 drops is sufficient to aromatically alter the spirit of a
room to suit the needs and desires of the
sensuous woman.

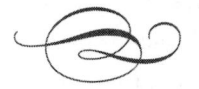

Relaxing Fragrances

Aromatic Oil, Max. Drops/Oil burner

Cedarwood, 2–3

Chamomile, 3

Clary Sage, 1–2

Cypress, 3–4

Frankincense, 3–4

Jasmine, 3

Lavender, 4

Marjoram, 4

Neroli, 3

Rose, 3

Sandalwood, 4

Vetivert, 1–2

Ylang Ylang, 3

Uplifting Fragrances

Aromatic Oil, Max. Drops/Oil burner

Basil, 1–2

Bergamot, 4

Clary Sage, 1–2

Clove, 2

Geranium, 3

Grapefruit, 4

Jasmine, 3

Juniper, 4

Lemon, 5

Orange, 5

Patchouli, 1–2

Pine, 3

Rosemary, 4

Harmonizing Fragrances

Aromatic Oil, Max. Drops/Oil burner

Bergamot, 4

Cedarwood, 2–3

Frankincense, 3–4

Geranium, 3

Lavender, 4

Melissa, 4

Rose, 3

Stimulating Fragrances

Aromatic Oil, Max. Drops/Oil burner

Basil, 1–2

Black Pepper, 2–3

Clove, 2

Grapefruit, 4

Juniper, 4

Lemon, 5

Peppermint, 3

Rosemary, 4

Thyme, 3

Arousing Fragrances

Aromatic Oil, Max. Drops/Oil burner

Black Pepper, 2–3

Cedarwood, 2–3

Clary Sage, 1–2

Clove, 2

Jasmine, 3

Neroli, 3

Patchouli, 1–2

Pine, 3

Rose, 3

Sandalwood, 4

Vetivert, 1–2

Ylang Ylang, 3

The Fragrances
The Sensuous Woman's Guide to the Essential Oils and the Base Oils

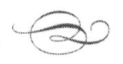

The following guide describes the unique personality and potentials of twenty-eight particularly lovely fragrances captured in their purest, most accessible form as essential oils. While the aromatic formulations presented throughout the book evoke many moods and meet many needs, personalized fragrances may also be created to express an individual essence or address a specific need. To facilitate the selection and enjoyment of an appropriate and appealing essential oil, the guide has classified each according to fragrance, effects on mood and emotion, and suggested uses in the special moments of every day.

Fragrance

The fragrance of each essential oil is categorized as *citrus, floral, herbal, menthol, musky, spicy,* or *woodland*. In addition, the intensity and persistence of the fragrance are described as *top notes* (light and fleeting aromas), *middle notes* (moderately intense and persistent aromas), and *base notes* (heavier and most long-lasting aromas). Suggestions for fragrances that blend well together are also listed.

Effects on Mood and Emotion

Each oil is described in terms of its overall effects as *relaxing, uplifting, harmonizing, stimulating,* and *arousing*.

Suggested Uses

An essential oil may be used alone or combined with two to three other oils, each chosen to evoke a desired effect on the mind and emotions and, of course, to delight the senses with its beautiful aroma. Before use, the essential oils must always be diluted in water or a vegetable base oil (see pages 177–184) or commercial unscented lotion. The recommended maximum number of drops that may be added to the bath, facial oils, body lotions, perfumes, or air fragrancers is provided for each essential oil in the guide.

Cautions

The essential oils are pure, powerful products of nature and any specific cautions are noted where necessary. As a general caveat, however, the oils are not intended for internal use and contact with the eyes should be avoided. If, despite following the guidelines, skin irritation or tingling develops, the affected area may be rubbed with a vegetable oil, such as sweet almond or olive oil, until the reaction subsides, usually within an hour.

Storage

If stored in dark glass bottles away from heat and light and if tightly closed after each use, most essential oils last for at least six months.

• • •

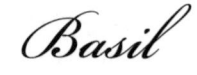

Basil

The name of this fragrant herb is derived from the Greek *basilikon*, meaning "royal," and indeed basil is an ideal anointment for a king. The rich, penetrating scent of basil not only helps combat mental fatigue but increases concentration, improves memory, and paves the way for decisive action. This aromatic herb with soft, broad, oval leaves, small white flowers, and long, leafy stalks is considered a sacred plant in India, where it is called *tulsi*. Dedicated to the Hindu gods Vishnu and Krishna, the herb is sometimes chewed before religious ceremonies, presumably to prepare the mind for introspection. Although cultivated for at least 4,000 years in Asia where it is indigenous, basil was introduced to Europe only in the Middle Ages. Here it was renowned as a nerve tonic and recommended by the famous sixteenth-century herbalist John Gerard to "taketh away sorrowfulness" and "maketh a man merrie and glad." A popular strewing herb in England, basil was scattered on the floor to give off fragrance when stepped on, or powdered into snuff to relieve fainting and hysteria. Basil is one of a select group of essential oils used for sharpening the mind while steadying the emotions—characteristics necessary for any leader, whether of royal lineage or not.

Fragrance

Herbal

This pale yellow-green oil has a clear, refreshing characteristic scent that is spicy-sweet and slightly camphorous. A pleasing top note, basil oil blends well with bergamot, geranium, and lavender.

Effects on Mood and Emotion

Basil calms and tranquilizes as well as elevates the spirits during times of stress or sadness. If these states are accompanied by insomnia with persistent anxious thoughts, basil—particularly if combined with lavender—helps to clear the mind for restful sleep. The fragrance is known to strengthen the mental faculties of concentration and memory and to help resolve the uncomfortable states of indecision and confusion. The result is a feeling of renewed vigor and vitality and the determination to act rather than react to life's challenges.

Suggested Uses

The energizing fragrance of basil oil may be enjoyed in the bath as an uplifting start to the day or as a rejuvenating break before a social evening. The oil is also excellent in massage blends to strengthen and tone the muscles while invigorating the mind. Just one or two drops of this powerful oil burned in a room fragrancer is sufficient to inspire a firm sense of resolve and calm concentration. But if the scent proves too strong, a lighter fragrance such as geranium may be added to soften the aroma without hindering the effect.

Caution

Avoid during pregnancy. Use as recommended to prevent possible tingling or irritation of the skin.

Sensuous Pleasures

Basil
An Uplifting and Stimulating fragrance

Uses, Max. Drops

Bath oil, 2–3 in full bath

Body lotion, 3/1 Tbsp. base oil*

Perfume, 2/1 Tbsp. jojoba oil

Air fragrance, 1–2 in oil burner

*Equivalent to one handful of base oil

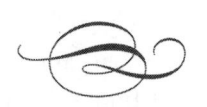

Bergamot

The smallest and most delicate of the citrus trees, bergamot was brought to Europe by Christopher Columbus, who discovered it growing in the Canary Islands. Probably native to tropical Asia, this lovely little tree has lush green oval leaves and star-shaped fragrant white flowers with oblong petals. Bergamot bears an inedible pear-shaped fruit with a thin, pale-yellow rind from which the essence is extracted. The tree is said to be named either after the Italian city of Bergamo in Lombardy where the fragrance was apparently first sold, or derived from the Turkish *begarmundi* (bey's pear) to describe the fruit's shape.

Fragrance

Citrus

This light, emerald-green oil has a warm, slightly spicy citrus scent. Lively, refreshing, with a delicate floral undertone, bergamot is a favorite top note in many fine perfumes, including the classic eau de cologne. The essence blends well with most other aromatic oils, especially black pepper, chamomile, cypress, frankincense, geranium, jasmine, juniper, lavender, neroli, orange, patchouli, rose, rosemary, sandalwood, and ylang ylang.

Effects on Mood and Emotion

The essence of bergamot is both uplifting and calming, depending on personal need, making it a truly harmonizing fragrance, especially when there is fear, anxiety, grief, depression, or nervous agitation. If the way ahead is unclear or uncertain, this versatile oil is also said to help restore clarity, perspective, and confidence.

Suggested Uses

One of the most beautiful and harmonizing of the essential oils, bergamot is uniquely appropriate when the emotional effects of stress or depression are echoed in the physical body. The oil may be used in many pleasurable ways: as an uplifting bath, especially when combined with geranium and lavender (2 drops of each); as a soothing and reassuring massage oil; as a gently feminine perfume; or as a delicate air fragrance to lighten the mood.

Caution

Bergamot increases photosensitivity and should therefore be avoided before exposure to the sun or other sources of ultraviolet light. Use as recommended to prevent possible tingling or irritation of the skin.

• • •

Citrus Oils

Bergamot

Grapefruit

Lemon

Orange

Bergamot
An Uplifting and Harmonizing fragrance

Uses, Max. Drops

Bath oil, 2–3 in full bath

Body lotion, 3/1 Tbsp. base oil*

Perfume, 8/1 Tbsp. jojoba oil

Air fragrance, 4 in oil burner

Equivalent to one handful of base oil

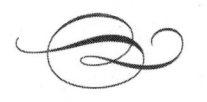

Black Pepper

Black pepper is indigenous to the low, damp forests of Asia, particularly southern India and Indonesia, and in fact its name is probably derived from the Sanskrit *pippali*, later changed to the Latin *piper*. One of the oldest known spices along with cinnamon and clove, black pepper has been used for culinary and medicinal purposes for over 4,000 years in the Far East and since at least the fifth century in Europe. In antiquity, black pepper was generally regarded as more valuable than gold, and Attila the Hun is said to have demanded 3,000 pounds of pepper as part of the ransom of Rome. Less well-recognized but no less precious than its use as a spice is the use of black pepper for its warm and stimulating fragrance. The aromatic oil is distilled from the dried, crushed, still unripe berries or peppercorns of the pepper plant, a climbing perennial vinelike shrub with a thick, round, woody stem, dark green heart-shaped leaves, and small white flowers that bear fruit on elongated, spiky offshoots. Originally a woodland species, the pepper plant may grow to more than twenty feet under natural conditions and must cling to nearby trees for support and shade. The vines bear fruit only after two to three years of growth but may continue to produce for up to twenty years.

Fragrance

Spicy

The pale amber essential oil of black pepper turns darker and thicker with age. Its scent is similarly dark and mysterious, with a spicy, hot, pungent aroma. A warm middle note, black pepper oil blends well with the citrus oils, cedarwood, frankincense, jasmine, juniper, rosemary, sandalwood, and ylang ylang.

Effects on Mood and Emotion

Ruled by Mars, black pepper is a strengthener and a stimulant with a somewhat masculine undertone that helps promote stamina, build courage, sharpen concentration, and enhance sexual prowess. It is also said that the natural warming qualities of the fragrance give comfort to a heart made cold by sorrow or neglect.

Suggested Uses

Black pepper is a gentle mental and physical stimulant and is thus excellent in massage blends designed to increase physical stamina or revive energy following arduous activity. The warm and dusky sensuality of black pepper oil is also a wonderful addition to a romantic evening, whether used as an enticing perfume, a subtly seductive fragrance in the air, or an exotic bath for two.

Caution

Use as recommended to prevent local redness and irritation of the skin.

Sensuous Pleasures

Black Pepper
A Stimulating and Arousing fragrance

Uses, Max. Drops

Bath oil, 2–3 in full bath

Body lotion, 3/1 Tbsp. base oil*

Perfume, 3–4/1 Tbsp. jojoba oil

Air fragrance, 2–3 in oil burner

*Equivalent to one handful of base oil

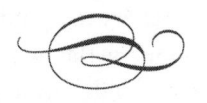

Cedarwood

One of the oldest aromatics, cedarwood oil was highly valued by the ancient Egyptians, who employed it in all facets of life: as a cosmetic, hair tonic, perfume, incense, medicine, and embalming potion. Prized as a building wood because of its hardness, durability, and ability to repel insects, the Egyptians used cedarwood in the construction of sarcophagi, temple doors, ship's masts, furniture, and jewelry. Even papyrus leaves were soaked in cedarwood oil to protect them from decay. Vast quantities of cedarwood were later used to build King Solomon's temple in Jerusalem or burned as incense during religious festivals. Further east, in Mesopotamia, frankincense, myrrh, cypress, and cedarwood were mixed with mortar to ensure that the holy shrines exuded a heavenly scent in the heat of the sun. The tree was considered a symbol of constant faith by the early Israelites, and its imagery is found in the Old Testament as a metaphor for the majesty, abundance, and richness of God's gifts to man. The oil was originally distilled from the cedar of Lebanon (*Cedrus libani*), which for centuries thrived in huge "holy forests" and of which only a few hundred now survive. A pyramid-shaped evergreen with bunches of needles on widely projecting branches and upright barrel-like cones, this stately tree may live for thousands of years. The essential oil of cedarwood that is available today comes primarily from two sources: the Atlas or Atlantic cedar (*Cedrus atlantica*), which is a close relative of the Lebanon cedar; and the Virginian or Red cedar

(*Juniperus virginiana*), which is a juniper and not a true cedar tree. The fragrance of cedarwood oil, like its majestic parent, inspires a sense of awe and promotes spiritual strength and inner calm.

Fragrance
Woodland
The thick, syrupy, golden oil of cedarwood has a rich, woody scent that is somewhat masculine in its warm, deep undertone. A pleasant base note in perfumes, cedarwood oil blends well with the citrus oils, black pepper, clary sage, cypress, frankincense, jasmine, juniper, lavender, melissa, neroli, pine, rose, rosemary, and sandalwood.

Effects on Mood and Emotion
The fragrance of cedarwood harmonizes the mind, body, and spirit and helps relax an over-intellectualized mind. The wood has been burned for millennia as incense to increase spiritual awareness while solidly grounding the believer in the here and now. The resultant combination of inner quiet and firm belief is especially beneficial for those lacking in confidence or self-esteem. Cedarwood oil is thus a marvelous strengthening tonic for encouraging self-acceptance, self-love, and—as an added benefit—sensuality and sexual pleasure.

Suggested Uses
During the 1800s women saturated handkerchiefs with cedarwood oil to inhale the scent in moments of duress. The oil may still be used in this way or vaporized in the air when a calm, confident sense of self is sorely needed. The enticing warmth of cedarwood may also be combined with other sen-

sual fragrances such as jasmine and neroli for a romantic bath (2 drops of each) or a truly sensational massage blend (2 drops of each/1 tablespoon of base oil). Egyptian women combed cedarwood oil in their hair to encourage growth, and indeed the oil is ideal as a hair rinse to add luster and allure, especially to dark hair.

Caution
Avoid during pregnancy. Use as recommended to prevent possible tingling or irritation of the skin.

Sensuous Pleasures

Cedarwood
A Relaxing, Harmonizing, and Arousing fragrance

Uses, Max. Drops

Bath oil, 2–3 in full bath

Body lotion, 3/1 Tbsp. base oil*

Perfume, 6/1 Tbsp. jojoba oil

Air fragrance, 2–3 in oil burner

Equivalent to one handful of base oil

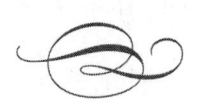

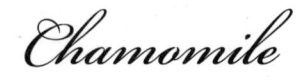

Chamomile

The ancient Egyptians considered chamomile a sacred flower and dedicated it to the sun god, Ra. Chamomile in turn worships the sun, opening its delicate white flowers to the light and closing them again in the dark. The plant is part of the prolific Asteraceae botanical family, which includes more than 13,000 plant species growing in temperate climates around the world. There are numerous varieties of this herbaceous perennial, all of which resemble the daisy with flowers of white petals and gold centers, a slender, hairy stalk, and fine feathery leaves. Roman chamomile (*Chamaemelum nobile*), also known as sweet or English chamomile, is indigenous to England, where it blooms throughout the summer from June to August. It was known to the early Saxons as "maythem" and was considered one of their most precious herbs. In Elizabethan times the flowers, which yield their scent when crushed, were woven into turf seats, planted along garden paths, nurtured as well-trimmed chamomile lawns or strewn across household floors. Chamomile has been called the "plant's physician" because of its ability to keep surrounding plants healthy—and is perhaps one of the gentlest and most healing of the aromatic oils.

Fragrance

Herbal

Always influenced by the light, the pale blue aromatic oil of chamomile becomes greenish yellow on exposure. The oil has a refreshing fruity fragrance reminiscent of apples, which gave rise to its Greek name, *kamai melon* or ground apples. A pleasing middle note, chamomile blends well with the citrus oils, geranium, lavender, neroli, sandalwood, and rose.

Effects on Mood and Emotion

For hypersensitivity or irritability from whatever cause—anger, melancholy, anxiety—chamomile acts as a soothing and calming balm. The gentle sedative effects of its fragrance were known to Egyptian priests and English country folk alike who used chamomile to promote a sense of inner balance, peacefulness, and patience.

Suggested Uses

The lovely chamomile soothes oversensitivity and tension when used as a relaxing bath oil or massage blend. The oil has an affinity for healing dry, irritated skin and has been renowned since antiquity as a shampoo to lighten and enhance the beauty of fair hair. In a perfume or air fragrancer, chamomile inspires the centeredness that is a necessary prerequisite to all connectedness.

Sensuous Pleasures

Chamomile
A Relaxing fragrance

Uses, Max. Drops

Bath oil, 2–3 in full bath

Facial oil, 2/1 Tbsp. base oil*

Body lotion, 3/1 Tbsp. base oil**

Perfume, 2/1 Tbsp. jojoba oil

Air fragrance, 3 in oil burner

Roughly one month's supply
**Equivalent to one handful of base oil*

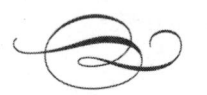

Clary Sage

Clary sage oil is derived from the herbaceous biennial or perennial also known as meadow sage due to its predilection for sunny, open spaces. Not to be confused with common or garden sage, this dramatic plant may reach as high as two or three feet, and rests on a square sturdy stalk with large velvety heart-shaped leaves. The plant's small purple or white flowers emerge from pointed green and lilac bracts that radiate out symmetrically from the reddish stalk. The overall effect is extravagant and evocative. Since the sixteenth century, clary sage has been used in the production of wine and beer, and indeed the fragrance can cause an intoxicating sense of euphoria and relaxation.

Fragrance

Herbal

The aroma of this clear essential oil is elevating and invigorating. Nutty, strong, slightly musky, and sensual, clary sage adds a unique middle note that blends well with cedarwood, the citrus oils, frankincense, geranium, jasmine, juniper, lavender, melissa, rose, rosemary, and sandalwood.

Effects on Mood and Emotion

Clary sage is both a relaxing and an uplifting essential oil that helps lighten the heavy states of fatigue, sadness, or fear. The oil is said to reawaken the weary, soothe the despondent, and calm the anxious. The fragrance of clary sage inspires dreams, stimulates creativity, and sets free the spirit for passion.

Suggested Uses

When used in the bath, massaged on the body, worn as a perfume or wafted through the air, the slightly musky, freely sensuous fragrance of clary sage creates a mood of excitement verging on elation, combined with a deep-seated sense of relaxed well-being. The oil is also an effective moisturizer for dry or mature skin as well as an astringent and gentle cleanser for oily skin.

Caution

Avoid during pregnancy. Not recommended before driving or in conjunction with even small amounts of alcohol.

Clary Sage

**A Relaxing, Uplifting, and
Arousing fragrance**

Uses, Max. Drops

Bath oil, 2 in full bath

Facial oil, 1/1 Tbsp. base oil*

Body lotion, 3/1 Tbsp. base oil**

Perfume, 6/1 Tbsp. jojoba oil

Air fragrance, 1–2 in oil burner

Roughly one month's supply
**Equivalent to one handful of base oil*

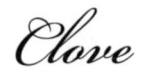

Clove

The Portuguese navigator Vasco da Gama is reported to have discovered the clove tree growing in the tropical Molucca Islands—or Spice Islands—of Indonesia during his voyages there in the fifteenth century. The Portuguese retained almost exclusive rights to its valuable trade for roughly 200 years until invasion by the Dutch, who apparently destroyed all clove plantations save one to better secure a monopoly. This was eventually broken by the French, who are said to have stolen several Dutch plants for cultivation in their far-flung territories. The tree was then transported to other tropical climates by the English, who brought it to Malaysia, and finally by the Arabs, who cultivated clove in Zanzibar and the Pemba Islands of Tanzania during the early nineteenth century. The clove tree is a highly aromatic columnar evergreen, growing naturally to a height of thirty feet or more. The trunk, which has a smooth, grayish bark, divides into large branches with oblong leaves and brilliant crimson flowers. The essence of clove is extracted from the unopened flower buds once they have turned from green to rosy pink. The buds are harvested by hand or by beating the tree and are dried in the sun or gently heated for several days until they become the characteristic ruddy brown. The name "clove" is derived from the Latin *clavus*, meaning nail, which aptly describes the dried bud.

Fragrance

Spicy

Colorless to slightly yellow when first distilled, the aromatic oil becomes dark brown with maturity. A hot, penetrating, and spicy fragrance, clove oil is a distinctive base note that blends well with lighter fragrances, such as the citrus oils.

Effects on Mood and Emotion

Clove oil has a stimulating and uplifting quality that is reputed to strengthen the mind, especially the memory. The fragrance is therefore useful when there is weakness, lethargy, or depression, especially if due to loss or the inability to let go and move forward. Its warming, stimulating properties make clove oil a favorite in Eastern love potions.

Suggested Uses

Just a few drops of clove in an oil burner adds an enlivening, positive atmosphere to a room. The oil is particularly effective for the office as it helps focus concentration, or for the bedroom to stir romance. Clove's ability to purify the air in times of sickness is legendary, and it is said that when the Dutch destroyed the vast clove plantations of the Molucca Islands, outbreaks of disease reached epidemic proportions.

Caution

Avoid during pregnancy. Clove oil can cause irritation of the skin and is therefore not recommended for use in the bath or in skin preparations.

Sensuous Pleasures

Clove
A Uplifting, Stimulating,
and Arousing fragrance

Uses, Max. Drops

Air fragrance, 2 in oil burner

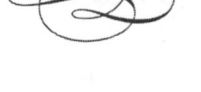

Cypress

Cypress (*Cupressus sempervirens*) lives forever — or so the cypress tree appears, with its evergreen leaves and durable wood seemingly immune to time. According to Greek mythology, Cyparissos was so distressed to have killed the sacred stag of his friend Apollo that he asked the gods to allow his grief to last forever, a wish they granted by turning him into a cypress tree. The ancient Egyptians, the Greeks, and the Romans all dedicated the tree to their gods of death, and for thousands of years the cypress has been planted in burial grounds and cemeteries. In some parts of the world, cypress branches are still hung in the home of the deceased or carried by mourners in funeral processions. Over time, however, the cypress as a symbol of grief and death was transformed into a symbol of the immortal soul and the spirit everlasting. This tall, conical perennial provided the wood for Egyptian sarcophagi, Greek sculpture, Phoenician ships and, if legend is correct, the cross of Christ. Not surprisingly, cypress contains abundant aromatic oil that is said to comfort the grieving.

Fragrance

Woodland

A favorite essence of the Assyrians, this pale yellow aromatic oil has a rich, woody fragrance reminiscent of pine needles. A warm and soft middle note, cypress oil blends well with cedarwood, the citrus oils, clary sage, juniper, lavender, pine, rosemary, and sandalwood.

Effects on Mood and Emotion

Cypress oil comforts and calms the distressed, especially in times of grief or transition. Like its parent, the cypress tree, the fragrance of the essential oil provides a sense of solace—soothing anger and anxiety and allowing for a restful sleep.

Suggested Uses

As the essential oil of cypress helps to overcome a sense of loss on an emotional level, so too does it control the loss of tone or loss of moisture on a physical level. In this capacity, cypress oil may be used in massage blends intended to gently tone the muscles of the body, from the breasts to the thighs and buttocks. The oil is also a valuable astringent for oily skin, as well as a soothing facial tonic for dehydrated or mature skin that has lost its fluid elasticity. The fragrance was highly valued as a soothing incense by the ancient civilizations and is known to have been a favorite of Hippocrates.

Caution

Avoid during pregnancy.

Sensuous Pleasures

Cypress
A Relaxing fragrance

Uses, Max. Drops

Bath oil, 4 in full bath

Facial oil, 2/1 Tbsp. base oil*

Body lotion, 4/1 Tbsp. base oil**

Perfume, 4–5/1 Tbsp. jojoba oil

Air fragrance, 3–4 in oil burner

*Roughly one month's supply
**Equivalent to one handful of base oil

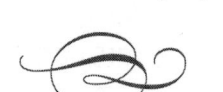

Frankincense

The scent of frankincense is elevating, inspiring, and conducive to prayer. For this reason it has always been regarded as a precious substance by those cultures steeped in a quest for the spiritual. The ancient Egyptians and Hebrews burned frankincense resin in religious ceremonies more than 5,000 years ago, and King Solomon is said to have spent a fortune securing its trade with the Queen of Somalia. So precious and so powerful were its spiritual effects that frankincense was one of the three gifts from the Magi to the baby Jesus. Both the incense and the aromatic oil of frankincense are obtained from the large drops or "tears" of milky resin that exude from the bark of a small gum tree of the *Boswellia* genus, most commonly *Boswellia carteri*. Despite its typically desert habitat, this magical plant produces abundant leaves and pale pink or white flowers.

Fragrance
Musky

Ruled by the sun, frankincense is a beautiful golden oil with a more subtle fragrance than the resin. Earthy and warm with a slight lemon scent, the oil has a mysterious, haunting quality. A deep base note, frankincense blends well with almost any scent, particularly black pepper, the citrus oils, geranium, jasmine, lavender, neroli, rose, sandalwood, and vetivert.

Effects on Mood and Emotion

The comforting scent of frankincense gently soothes and fortifies while helping to liberate the emotions from past grievances or fears. In freeing the spirit from negativity, frankincense oil also profoundly elevates the psyche, encouraging a search for the eternal and strengthening a connection with the divine. A truly harmonizing oil, frankincense deepens and slows the breathing, producing feelings of inner calm so helpful for prayer or meditation.

Suggested Uses

The Roman poet Ovid, in his treatise *Medicamina Faciei*, described frankincense as an excellent preparation for beautifying the face. The resin was also a particular favorite of the Egyptians, who used it in unguents and face masks for its firming and rejuvenating properties. Today, frankincense is considered the oil par excellence for mature skin as it helps to tone the skin and smooth away wrinkles. A gentle but powerful astringent, frankincense is also beneficial for oily skin. In an air fragrancer or as a perfume, frankincense lends a lingering aura of the mystical and the sublime. When combined with neroli and rose, the effect is truly stunning and exotic whether used in a bath (2 drops of each) or a massage blend (2 drops of each in 1 tablespoon base oil).

Frankincense
A Relaxing and Harmonizing fragrance

Uses, Max. Drops

Bath oil, 5–6 in full bath

Facial oil, 3/1 Tbsp. base oil*

Body lotion, 6/1 Tbsp. base oil**

Perfume, 6/1 Tbsp. jojoba oil

Air fragrance, 3–4 in oil burner

Roughly one month's supply

**Equivalent to one handful of base oil*

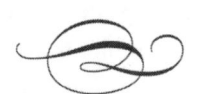

Geranium

According to Islamic folklore, the geranium was a gift from Allah to his prophet Mohammed—a generous gift as geranium oil is one of the loveliest and most versatile of the plant essences. It is derived not from the popular and familiar geranium often seen overflowing window boxes or hanging baskets but from the prolific *Pelargonium* species, of which *P. graveolens* and *P. odorantissimus* are most commonly distilled for their oil. This small fragrant plant has deeply lobed green leaves, rose-pink flowers that bloom at the end of terminal umbels, and beaklike fruits for which the plant was named by the Greeks as *geranion* or crane.

Fragrance

Floral

Lightly tinged with green, geranium oil has a sweet, fresh, floral scent resembling rose that aptly reflects the beauty and harmony normally associated with its ruling planet, Venus. A calming middle note, geranium oil blends well with most other fragrances, especially basil, the citrus oils, frankincense, jasmine, juniper, lavender, marjoram, neroli, rose, rosemary, and sandalwood.

Effects on Mood and Emotion

A balancing oil that helps to regulate the natural rhythms of the emotions, geranium may have either a calming or an uplifting effect, depending on individual need. It is thus very useful for anxiety states, depression, and debility, where the goal is equilibrium.

Suggested Uses

As a natural balancer, geranium oil is marvelous in facial oils for normal, dry, or oily skin, as well as for bringing a radiant and refreshing glow to mature faces. Its delightful aroma, when rinsed through the hair or worn as a perfume, conveys a charming and alluring femininity. Lovely and reviving, geranium may also be enjoyed in the bath or as a lingering fragrance in the air to quiet a room and keep the "evil spirits" at bay.

Sensuous Pleasures

Geranium
An Uplifting and Harmonizing fragrance

Uses, Max. Drops

Bath oil, 3–4 in full bath

Facial oil, 2/1 Tbsp. base oil*

Body lotion, 3/1 Tbsp. base oil**

Perfume, 4/1 Tbsp. jojoba oil

Air fragrance, 3 in oil burner

Roughly one month's supply
**Equivalent to one handful of base oil*

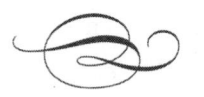

Grapefruit

A cultivated citrus tree with glossy green leaves, white flowers, and large, pendulous yellow fruit, the grapefruit is often used as an ornamental plant to beautify the gardens of the Mediterranean. The light, refreshing oil distilled from the fresh rind of the fruit is similarly a most useful aromatic oil for personal beauty care. A lovely oil, the aroma of grapefruit reverberates with sunshine and renews a zest for life.

Fragrance

Citrus

The yellowish-green essence of grapefruit has a light, fresh, fruity, and slightly sharp scent that as a lively top note blends well with basil, black pepper, cedarwood, clary sage, cypress, frankincense, geranium, lavender, orange, rosemary, sandalwood, thyme, and ylang ylang.

Effects on Mood and Emotion

The fragrance of grapefruit revitalizes and revives when energy is low or the emotions ponderous. A gentle, uplifting tonic, the fragrance of grapefruit helps counterbalance the effects of stress and stabilize mental states.

Suggested Uses

Grapefruit is an uplifting way to start the day either in a morning bath or in an air fragrancer to scatter the cobwebs of the night. The oil is said to stimulate the appetite and its aroma in the air is a most pleasing addition to any mealtime celebration.

Caution

Grapefruit increases photosensitivity and should therefore be avoided before exposure to the sun or other sources of ultraviolet light. Use as recommended to prevent tingling or irritation of the skin.

Sensuous Pleasures

Grapefruit
An Uplifting and Stimulating fragrance

Uses, Max. Drops

Bath oil, 3–4 in full bath

Body lotion, 3/1 Tbsp. base oil*

Perfume, 6/1 Tbsp. jojoba oil

Air fragrance, 4 in oil burner

*Equivalent to one handful of base oil

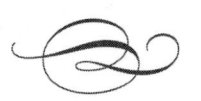

Jasmine

Jasmine is a fragrance of pure sensuality — a sensuality that transcends the physical and inspires the commingling of true lovers. Revered for thousands of years in the East as an integral part of the ritual and art of lovemaking, jasmine is still regarded as one of the greatest aphrodisiacs among the aromatic oils. This exquisite, fragrant oil has both a warm, unfolding quality that is quintessentially feminine as well as a deep, rich, powerful aspect that is clearly masculine, giving rise to its title "the king of essential oils." The botanical family includes several hundred species, two of which — *Jasminium officinale* and the large-blossomed *Jasminium grandiflorum* — are most commonly used for their aromatic oil in the West. The beautiful white flowers of this climbing tree are picked at night, when their aroma is most intense. Huge quantities of fresh flowers are needed to produce pure jasmine oil: 8 million hand-picked jasmine flowers yield roughly two pounds of oil, making this "oil of romance" also one of the most costly.

Fragrance

Floral

The oil is heavy, viscous, and a dark-hued reddish brown, but its aroma is light: sweet, heady, and heavenly. The Hindu god of love, Kama, is said to have pierced the hearts of lovers with a jasmine-scented arrow, and indeed the fragrance is almost irresistibly romantic. One of the "noble" oils of perfumery along with rose and neroli, jasmine is a stirring base note that blends well with black pepper, the citrus oils, geranium, lavender, neroli, rose, sandalwood, and ylang ylang.

Effects on Mood and Emotion

Jasmine has a profound effect on the emotions, inviting relaxation, clearing away worry, and calming the nerves. It is also a firmly uplifting fragrance that helps to counteract even severe melancholy and to instill positive feelings of confidence and optimism. But perhaps the most characteristic reaction to jasmine is a sublime arousal, not only of passion, but of yearnings for creativity and release from restraint.

Suggested Uses

The sails of Cleopatra's barge were soaked in jasmine to further the seduction of Mark Antony, and indeed the fragrance, when wafted through the air, sets a captivating mood of relaxed romance. The odalisques of the harem prepared themselves for the sultan by bathing in jasmine, oiling their hair, their bodies, and their lips with the sensual scent. The oil is said to be effective in increasing fertility in men and reducing emotionally related sexual problems and is thus a wise choice in massage blends for the sultan of any house.

Caution

Avoid during pregnancy.

•   •   •

Aromatic Aphrodisiacs

Black Pepper

Cedarwood

Clary Sage

Clove

Jasmine

Neroli

Patchouli

Pine

Rose

Sandalwood

Vetivert

Ylang Ylang

Sensuous Pleasures

Jasmine
A Relaxing, Uplifting, and Arousing fragrance

Uses, Max. Drops

Bath oil, 3 in full bath

Facial oil, 2/1 Tbsp. base oil*

Body lotion, 3/1 Tbsp. base oil**

Perfume, 3–4/1 Tbsp. jojoba oil

Air fragrance, 3 in oil burner

*Roughly one month's supply
**Equivalent to one handful of base oil*

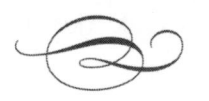

Juniper Berry

According to the folklore of many cultures, juniper has magical properties of protection. In medieval times, the berries were burned to drive out ghosts, or the green branches smoked to protect the farmer's crops and livestock. Perhaps it is no coincidence that the Virgin Mary and her baby Jesus are said to have sheltered from Herod's soldiers under a juniper bush. The essential oil of juniper is similarly considered to have a protective and purifying action, cleansing the spirit and ridding the body of toxins. Derived from a small, unassuming evergreen shrub or tree, depending on its habitat, the hardy juniper grows well in poor, arid soil. Its flowers are small and lemon yellow, blooming in the early summer. The fruit or berries are well hidden among the juniper's needlelike leaves and turn from green to blue-black as they gradually ripen over several years. The trees are unisexual, and a female juniper requires fertilization by a male tree in order to flower. Juniper is an ancient, enduring species: berries have been found in prehistoric dwellings, attesting to the plant's capacity for self-protection and renewal.

Fragrance

Woodland

The aromatic oil of juniper is colorless or pale yellow with a hint of green. The scent is fresh, balsamic, and reminiscent of the outdoors. A soft, warm middle note, juniper blends well with black pepper, the citrus oils, clary sage, cypress, frank-incense, geranium, lavender, pine, rosemary, and sandalwood.

Effects on Mood and Emotion

Juniper elevates the emotions from the heaviness of mental fatigue or anxiety, especially if due to a challenging situation, unpleasant event, or drain-ing personal attachment. When the mind needs to be strengthened and cleansed of unwanted feel-ings, the fragrance of juniper gently purifies and allows clear sight and renewed harmony.

Suggested Uses

The fresh, inspiring fragrance of juniper increases inner confidence when courage is necessary to combat fear and inhibition. It is thus a thoroughly uplifting fragrance whether used in the bath, vaporized in the air, massaged on the skin, or applied as perfume. The oil is also a valuable anti-septic for oily skin and is renowned for its detoxi-fying action when burned in a room during times of physical illness or emotional upset.

Caution

Avoid during pregnancy, or if there is kidney inflammation or disease.

Sensuous Pleasures

Juniper
An Uplifting and Stimulating fragrance

Uses, Max. Drops

Bath oil, 4 in full bath

Facial oil, 1/1 Tbsp. base oil*

Body lotion, 4/1 Tbsp. base oil**

Perfume, 5/1 Tbsp. jojoba oil

Air fragrance, 4 in oil burner

Roughly one month's supply
**Equivalent to one handful of base oil*

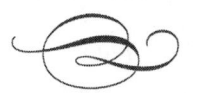

Lavender

While other plants have fallen out of favor, lavender has remained popular for thousands of years. This is perhaps due to its remarkable healing properties and unparalleled versatility, both as a remedy for physical and psychological disorders as well as a classic ingredient in fine perfumes and cosmetics. Native to Persia and the sun-drenched slopes of Mediterranean mountainsides, lavender was brought to the rest of Europe by the conquering Romans. Several varieties of lavender are cultivated for their aromatic oil, of which *Lavandula angustifolia* is the most delicately scented. The subtle, tiny mauve flowers of lavender bloom at the top of long, slender stems with narrow, silvery leaves. The flowers, stems, and leaves are covered with small star-shaped hairs that contain the oil glands, making the entire plant highly aromatic.

Fragrance

Floral

Lavender oil varies in color from clear to dark yellow or green. Its aroma is clean, fresh, floral, and light. A lively middle note, lavender has been a favorite component of perfumes for centuries, especially among English ladies of the Elizabethan and Stuart ages. The oil's effects are usually enhanced by combination with other fragrances, and it blends well with the citrus oils, cedarwood, chamomile, cypress, frankincense, geranium, juniper, marjoram, neroli, peppermint, pine, rose, rosemary, sandalwood, and ylang ylang.

Effects on Mood and Emotion

Lavender induces a sense of peacefulness and integration. Known for its stabilizing effects, the oil was said to guard against the excesses of unbridled emotions and was thus sprinkled on the heads of young maidens to help preserve their chastity. The profound ability of the fragrance to calm, to soothe, and to ease agitation continues to make it a superb choice for mood swings, depression, anxiety, and insomnia.

Suggested Uses

Lavender was the preferred bath oil of the ancient Romans, from which its name is derived: *lavare*, to wash. A soothing and relaxing oil, lavender may be added to a nighttime bath, a foot bath, or a massage blend to relieve a tired body or tense mind. Lavender oil has exceptional regenerative properties and rapidly promotes the growth of new cells. It is thus used in facial oils for all skin types, as well as for healing raw, chapped hands. Renowned as one of the noble oils of perfumery, the scent of lavender conveys tranquility and poise.

Lavender
A Relaxing and Harmonizing fragrance

Uses, Max. Drops

Bath oil, 5–6 in full bath

Facial oil, 3/1 Tbsp. base oil*

Body lotion, 6/1 Tbsp. base oil**

Perfume, 7/1 Tbsp. jojoba oil

Air fragrance, 4 in oil burner

Roughly one month's supply
**Equivalent to one handful of base oil*

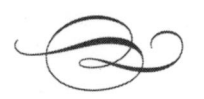

Lemon

Among the treasures brought back to Europe by the Crusaders in the early Middle Ages was the lovely lemon tree. This small, thorny evergreen has irregular branches and thick, shiny, oval leaves. Its white or pinkish fine-petaled flowers are beautifully fragranced, giving way to abundant acid fruit. The essence extracted from the rind of the still-green unripe fruit lifts the spirits, strengthens resolve, and builds vitality.

Fragrance

Citrus

A pale yellow or yellow-green color, lemon turns cloudy when exposed to sunlight. Its fragrance is clean and refreshing with the crisp zestiness of freshly cut lemons. A light top note, lemon blends well with bergamot, black pepper, chamomile, clary sage, cypress, frankincense, geranium, juniper, lavender, neroli, rosemary, sandalwood, and ylang ylang.

Effects on Mood and Emotion

In some early Christian art, the fruit depicted on the Tree of Knowledge is clearly a lemon. This is perhaps fitting as the oil is said to produce clarity of thinking and conciseness of expression. A reviving, cooling scent, lemon helps direct the focus when ideas are swirling in circles or when action is immobilized by indecision.

Suggested Uses

The fragrant lemon adds a touch of vivacity and youthful freshness to a perfume or air fragrance, while a few drops sprinkled in the bath energize and revitalize after even the hardest day. A renowned folk remedy, a few drops of lemon oil in an unperfumed shampoo or conditioner will naturally highlight fair hair.

Caution

Lemon increases photosensitivity and should therefore be avoided before exposure to the sun or other sources of ultraviolet light. Use as recommended to prevent possible tingling or irritation of the skin.

Sensuous Pleasures

Lemon
An Uplifting and Stimulating fragrance

Uses, Max. Drops

Bath oil, 1–2 in full bath

Body lotion, 2/1 Tbsp. base oil*

Perfume, 7/1 Tbsp. jojoba oil

Air fragrance, 5 in oil burner

Equivalent to one handful of base oil

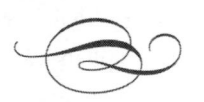

Marjoram

To the ancient Greeks, marjoram was a symbol of joy and good fortune and was said to have been given its fragrance following the touch of Aphrodite. The plant was therefore used to garland the heads of newlyweds or grown on gravesites to ensure contentment to the deceased. The Romans believed that marjoram engendered longevity, and it was one of the sacred herbs of India, dedicated to the gods Shiva and Vishnu. Above all else, this common culinary herb is warming and calming and is perhaps the most sedative of all the essential oils. Several varieties of marjoram are distilled for their oil: *Origanum marjorana* or sweet marjoram is the most common, but *Thymus mastichina* or wild Spanish marjoram may also be used, although it is technically not a true marjoram but a member of the thyme family. Sweet marjoram is a bushy low-growing plant with creeping roots, reddish woody stems, and small, velvety, often purplish leaves that hide clusters of tiny white, pink, or lilac flowers. The plant thrives on sunny hillsides—as its Greek name, *oros ganus*, or joy of the mountain, implies—and is harvested in summer, just before full flowering, to obtain the most fragrant oil.

Fragrance

Herbal

In Old England, marjoram was used both as a strewing herb and in nosegays to dispel unpleasant odors with its clean, fresh smell. The aromatic oil varies in color from clear to yellow-green or amber and has a strong, warm, penetrating herbal scent. A distinctive middle note, marjoram oil blends well with bergamot, geranium, lavender, peppermint, and rosemary.

Effects on Mood and Emotion

One of the most calming of all the fragrant oils, women in ancient Greece are known to have rubbed marjoram on their heads as a tranquilizer. The oil sedates the senses and acts as a superb hypnotic to induce peaceful sleep. By forming a barrier to the onslaught of stimuli, marjoram allows the mind and emotions time to turn off and catch up. It is especially comforting to a grieving heart or to soothe free-floating fears and nameless loneliness. However, as the fragrance may also sedate the sensual impulses, it is best used in moderation unless celibacy is desired.

Suggested Uses

Whenever disquiet and tension are the problems, marjoram oil is the solution. In a bath, massage blend, perfume, or air fragrancer, the soothing, refined scent of this essential oil inspires a sense of quiet well-being.

Caution

Avoid during pregnancy.

Sensuous Pleasures

Marjoram
A Relaxing fragrance

Uses, Max. Drops

Bath oil, 5–6 in full bath
Body lotion, 6/1 Tbsp. base oil*
Perfume, 3/1 Tbsp. jojoba oil
Air fragrance, 4 in oil burner
*Equivalent to one handful of base oil

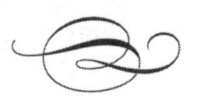

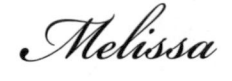

Melissa

Melissa is a bushy perennial herb with pale green serrated leaves and small white, yellow, or pale pink flowers. In southern Europe, where it originates, melissa is called heart's delight, perhaps because of its gentle appearance and sweet, endearing scent. The plant is named after the Greek mythological nymph Melissa, who was the protectress of bees. Irresistible to bees, melissa is traditionally planted in orchards to encourage pollination, or its leaves are crushed and placed on empty hives in spring to attract new swarms. Melissa is similarly enchanting as an aromatic oil with a fragrance that is youthful, cheering, and captivating. The ancient Greeks used melissa as a sedative, and Avicenna, the tenth-century Arab physician and philosopher, prized it for its calming and uplifting effects. Melissa oil is still used today as a gentle tonic to balance the emotions and set free the spirit for joy. As the yield of essential oil following distillation is extremely low, pure melissa oil is one of the most expensive aromatic oils, along with rose and jasmine, as well as one of the loveliest.

Fragrance

Citrus

Although not a citrus oil, melissa has a distinct lemony color and scent, but is more subtle than lemon oil. Delicate yet zesty, sweet yet provocative, fresh as a spring morning, melissa has an aroma as vivacious as a young girl. A slightly floral middle note, the oil blends well with many other essences including bergamot, cedarwood, clary sage, frankincense, geranium, lavender, neroli, rosemary, and ylang ylang.

Effects on Mood and Emotion

Like a flower opening to the honey bee, the fragrance of melissa helps open the heart to the joys of life. As such it has been used as an ancient remedy for melancholia and to comfort the grieving during times of loss. Melissa oil not only lifts the spirits but also soothes, sedates, and calms even the most extreme emotions. At the moment of greatest fear or despair, the fragrance of melissa oil helps pave the way to love, acceptance, forgiveness, and faith.

Suggested Uses

Melissa was one of the primary ingredients of a fourteenth-century perfume called Carmelite water, after the French Carmelite nuns who produced it. Although expensive, the oil adds a charming, sunny note to perfume blends and an uplifting, optimistic atmosphere when vaporized into the air. Melissa is considered a rejuvenating oil, perhaps because of its calming and liberating effects on the emotions.

Caution

Avoid during pregnancy. Use as recommended to prevent possible tingling or irritation of the skin.

Sensuous Pleasures

Melissa
A Harmonizing fragrance

Uses, Max. Drops

Bath oil, 2–3 in full bath
Body lotion, 3/1 Tbsp. base oil*
Perfume, 5/1 Tbsp. jojoba oil
Air fragrance, 4 in oil burner

*Equivalent to one handful of base oil

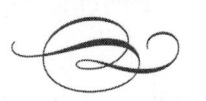

Neroli

Extracted from the intensely fragrant large white blossoms of the bitter orange tree known as *Citrus aurantium* or *Citrus bigaradia*, neroli is one of nature's most exquisite perfumes. The derivation of its name is somewhat controversial, although it is probably named after a fashionable sixteenth-century Italian perfume popularized by Anna Maria de la Tremoille, Princess of Neroli. The Princess is said to have used orange blossom oil so lavishly that even her gloves were scented with its fragrance. Neroli oil is still used today in the finest perfumes, including the true eau de cologne, and is certainly one of the most precious of the fragrant oils. Two thousand pounds of hand-picked orange blossoms yields only slightly more than two pounds of aromatic oil.

Fragrance

Floral

The aroma of neroli is unique, luxurious, sweet, and feminine—a haunting, tranquil scent. Clear or pale yellow in color, the oil turns reddish brown when exposed to light or air. A gorgeous floral base note, neroli blends well with most other oils, especially cedarwood, chamomile, the citrus oils, frankincense, geranium, jasmine, lavender, rose, rosemary, sandalwood, and vetivert.

Effects on Mood and Emotion

Neroli, with its joyful, inspiring scent, is one of the foremost tranquilizers among the essential oils. It was used in Victorian England to treat "the vapors" and is superb at subduing frantic emotions, such as anxiety with panic, sudden emotional shock with hysteria, or pacing, restless insomnia. The fragrance of neroli is also a mild aphrodisiac, probably due to its ability to allay fear. Appropriately, orange blossoms are woven into bridal bouquets and the flower has come to symbolize the purity of conjugal love.

Suggested Uses

This luxurious aromatic oil, renowned for its action on the skin, was used by Marie Antoinette to improve her complexion. Like geranium and lavender, neroli oil is good for all skin types, but especially for dry, sensitive, or even irritated skin. While all essential oils stimulate the regeneration of cells to some degree, lavender and neroli are particularly effective in this capacity, making the oil especially beneficial for mature skin. As a soothing bath oil, fragrant face lotion, sensual massage blend, sweetly scented hair rinse, or floral perfume, the fragrance of neroli exudes a graceful air of femininity and tranquility.

Neroli

A Relaxing and Arousing fragrance

Uses, Max. Drops

Bath oil, 3–4 in full bath

Facial unguent, 2/1 Tbsp. base oil*

Body lotion, 3–4/1 Tbsp. base oil**

Perfume, 4–5/1 Tbsp. jojoba oil

Air fragrance, 3 in oil burner

Roughly one month's supply

**Equivalent to one handful of base oil*

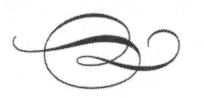

Orange

Three aromatic oils are derived from the orange tree: neroli from the large white blossoms; petitgrain oil from the oblong shiny leaves; and orange from the rind of the fruit. The fruit may take up to a year to fully form, and flowers and fruit may appear simultaneously on the same tree. Oranges are typically green when ripe and only turn orange when the temperature becomes cooler than their tropical norm. This versatile and abundant species yields a fruit that embodies the feelings of sunshine and good cheer, as does its fragrance. The "golden apple" awarded by Paris to Venus for her beauty and grown in the garden of Hesperides was most probably an orange, and until relatively recently it was given as a luxurious gift at Christmastime.

Fragrance

Citrus

The aroma of orange retains the zesty tang of the fresh fruit. Sweet, cheery, radiant, and refreshing, orange is a delicate top note that blends well with bergamot, black pepper, clary sage, clove, cypress, frankincense, geranium, grapefruit, juniper, neroli, patchouli, rosemary, sandalwood, vetivert, and ylang ylang. A deep golden-yellow in color, the oil can quickly turn brown and lose its pleasant aroma if exposed to the light.

Effects on Mood and Emotion

Like the refreshing lift from a sweet slice of orange, the fragrance raises the spirits, spreading a sense of light and optimism. A gentle boost on sad, heavy days, orange oil is also a mildly sedating relaxant during times of tension or fear.

Suggested Uses

The light, uplifting scent of orange makes an excellent addition to the morning bath, bringing a bit of sunshine to even the grayest day. Used in an oil burner, the fragrance imbues the atmosphere with a joyful, positive mood and is certainly one of the most delightful aromatic oils to waft through a dining room, especially on special occasions.

Caution

Orange increases photosensitivity and should therefore be avoided before exposure to the sun or other sources of ultraviolet light. Use as recommended to prevent possible tingling or irritation of the skin.

Orange
An Uplifting fragrance

Uses, Max. Drops

Bath oil, 3 in full bath

Body lotion, 3/1 Tbsp. base oil*

Perfume, 8/1 Tbsp. jojoba oil

Air fragrance, 5 in oil burner

*Equivalent to one handful of base oil

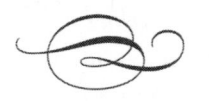

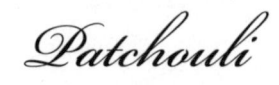

Patchouli

Apparently named after the Indian area of Pacholi, where fabrics and shawls were scented with dried patchouli leaves to repel moths before exportation to Europe, the fragrance became synonymous with "authentic" Indian cashmere during Victorian times. The oil is distilled from the broad, soft leaves of an egg-shaped herbaceous shrub with a square stem and white flowers. Patchouli has the unique characteristic of improving in fragrance over time, although even with age the scent is not universally appealing. Strong and earthy, more animal than floral in its aura, patchouli is known as a grounding oil. Good for dreamers, patchouli was a popular fragrance among the Flower Power generation of the 1960s.

Fragrance

Musky

The thick oil of patchouli is a deep ruby red, almost brown in color, with yellow or green highlights. The aroma is strong, musky, and persistent, making it an excellent fixative in perfumes. A penetrating base note that is best used sparingly, patchouli blends well with bergamot, frankincense, geranium, lavender, neroli, orange, pine, rose, and ylang ylang.

Effects on Mood and Emotion

This earthy, mildly sedating fragrance stimulates the desire for a sexual union that is uninhibited by societal conventions. The result is a calm, pervasive sense of individual powerfulness, which is enhanced by the oil's capacity to banish lethargy and sharpen the wits.

Suggested Uses

Provocative and sensual, patchouli has been used as an aphrodisiac for centuries. When added to the bath, combined into a body oil, worn as a perfume, or vaporized into the air, the effect of patchouli is frankly alluring. The oil is also advocated as a mild antiseptic for oily skin or to stimulate the growth of healthy new tissue in mature skin. Patchouli is said to promote skin toning, and is thus often recommended in massage blends.

Sensuous Pleasures

Patchouli
An Uplifting and Arousing fragrance

Uses, Max. Drops

Bath oil, 1–2 in full bath
Facial oil, 1/1 Tbsp. base oil*
Body lotion, 2/1 Tbsp. base oil**
Perfume, 4/1 Tbsp. jojoba oil
Air fragrance, 1–2 in oil burner

*Roughly one month's supply
**Equivalent to one handful of base oil

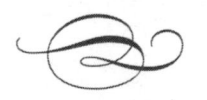

Peppermint

According to Greek mythology, Persephone became so jealous of her husband Pluto's affection for the young nymph Mentha that she ground the girl into the earth, whereupon Pluto, desiring to still enjoy the maiden, transformed her remains into the fragrant herb peppermint. This perennial plant with clusters of spiked lilac flowers and serrated leaves covered on their underside with fine hairs was known to many ancient civilizations. The Greeks and Romans garlanded their heads with peppermint during feasts—perhaps aware of its unparalleled capacity to relieve indigestion. Like Mentor, the wise guardian in the *Odyssey*, *Mentha x piperita*—peppermint—is one of a select group of aromatic oils known to increase intellectual prowess.

Fragrance

Menthol

Peppermint oil is colorless or pale yellow, but thickens and darkens with age. It has a lively, refreshing aroma with a characteristic menthol overtone. Used in small amounts so as not to overwhelm a blend, peppermint oil is a distinctive middle note that blends well with such fragrances as lavender, marjoram, and rosemary.

Effects on Mood and Emotion

The Roman author Pliny wrote that peppermint roused the conscious mind. Thousands of years later, the oil is still being used to strengthen the memory, focus concentration, and revive mental fatigue. The stimulating action of peppermint oil is similarly advocated to reverse states of emotional shock, especially if combined with nausea, faintness, trembling, or palpitations.

Suggested Uses

The cooling, refreshing fragrance of peppermint creates an energizing bath or delightful (and deodorizing) summer foot bath. The ancient Hebrews used peppermint as a perfume, and a few drops combined with compatible scents results in an uplifting, subtly stirring fragrance. A symbol of hospitality to the Romans, the aroma of peppermint in the air enhances the festivity of any occasion.

Caution

Avoid during pregnancy. Use as recommended to prevent possible tingling and irritation of the skin.

Sensuous Pleasures

Peppermint
A Stimulating fragrance

Uses, Max. Drops

Bath oil, 1–2 in full bath

Body lotion, 2/1 Tbsp. base oil*

Perfume, 2/1 Tbsp. jojoba oil

Air fragrance, 3 in oil burner

*Equivalent to one handful of base oil

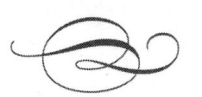

Pine

Said to be one of the few surviving trees of the Ice Age, the pine tree fares well in cold weather and is found in the mountainous regions of northern Europe. The tree has deeply fissured reddish-brown bark, gray-green needles, and sharp, pointed cones. Flowers of the male tree are yellow tinged with orange while those of the female tree are pink with a hint of green. The generic name *Pinus sylvestris* originates from the Latin word for tree, and indeed the evergreen pine is the embodiment of its species. Tall and powerful, the pine was considered a phallic symbol by the ancients, who believed the spirit of a fertility god had passed into the tree. As such, the pine has been used to represent passionate love, fecundity, and fidelity throughout the ages.

Fragrance

Like the forest from whence it comes, the aroma of pine is crisp, clear, and refreshing. The colorless or very pale yellow essential oil makes a slightly masculine middle note that blends well with cedarwood, lavender, lemon, patchouli, and rosemary.

Effects on Mood and Emotion

An ancient symbol of male virility, pine oil is an exhilarating aphrodisiac. The fragrance is equally effective for overcoming mental fatigue, nervous exhaustion, or general debility, and for promoting feelings of warm well-being.

Suggested Uses

Pine oil is a pleasing, naturally sensual scent that adds an uplifting romantic note when used in the bath, on the body, or as a unique perfume. A powerful antiseptic, the oil may also be vaporized to refresh the air before a romantic evening.

Caution

Use as recommended to prevent possible tingling or irritation of the skin.

Pine
An Uplifting and Arousing fragrance

Uses, Max. Drops

Bath oil, 2–3 in full bath
Body lotion, 3/1 Tbsp. base oil*
Perfume, 5/1 Tbsp. jojoba oil
Air fragrance, 3 in oil burner

*Equivalent to one handful of base oil

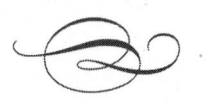

Rose

With its deep red velvety flower like the blood of Venus, the rose—the queen of flowers, the perfume of angels—surpasses all description of itself. An almost primeval symbol of perfect love and beauty, the rose was placed in the tombs of pharaohs to fragrance their journey to the afterlife, adorned the temples of Greece and Rome as an offering to the gods, and was considered by the early Christian mystics as the flower of Mary. It is said that Saint Dominic received a vision of the rosary from the Virgin Mary, and that each bead was scented with roses. The fragrance of the rose was first captured in its material form by the tenth-century physician and alchemist, Avicenna. In the process of mixing the flower with various metals in order to transmute them into gold, Avicenna extracted instead the fragrance of the flower in its concentrated essence. Of the 250 distinct species of roses, only two "old" roses are generally cultivated for their aromatic oil: *Rosa damascena*, the deep red damask or Bulgar rose, and *Rosa centifolia*, the highly fragrant pale pink cabbage rose. *R. damascena* is native to Persia and was brought to Europe by the returning Crusaders. Cultivated since the seventeenth century in the high Balkan mountains, Bulgaria remains the primary area of cultivation. While certainly exquisite, Bulgar rose is extremely rare and almost prohibitively expensive: thirty roses yield only one drop of rose essence; 60,000 roses produce one ounce. *R. centifolia*, which is considered equally

fragrant although not so rare, is therefore frequently distilled for its aromatic essence.

Fragrance

Floral

Perhaps the most feminine and seductive of fragrances, rose oil is the embodiment of perfume. As
a flawless base note, the oil blends well with bergamot, cedarwood, chamomile, clary sage, frankincense, geranium, jasmine, lavender, neroli,
patchouli, sandalwood, and ylang ylang. Rose
water made from an infusion of rose petals is a
gentle, light alternative to the more costly rose oil.

Effects on Mood and Emotion

The Romans scattered rose petals on the bridal
bed in much the same way as newlyweds today
are covered with rose-petal confetti. A symbol of
pure love and creativity, rose oil awakens a desire
for sensual pleasure in a characteristically womanly way: unfolding, yielding, tantalizing. The fragrance inspires a love that is universal: a love of
life, a joy in its beauty, and a sense of harmony
with the divine. The feminine, nurturing quality of
the fragrance is said to give solace to a heart broken by grief or remorse and to engender a confident feeling of well-being.

Suggested Uses

The rose was a favorite flower of the Romans,
who perfumed the streets with rose petals, scented
their fountains with roses, scattered roses from
the ceiling at ceremonial banquets, and flavored
their favorite food and wine with rose water. In
the home, clothes, bed linen, and cushions were
scented with roses; earthenware was soaked in

rose oil to imbue it with fragrance. Even the wings of birds were dotted with rose oil to perfume the air as they flew about a room. Roman women luxuriated in rose-fragranced baths and were massaged by slaves with rose oil. Their hair was rinsed with rose water, and their skin softened and revitalized with rose and honey facials. While the lavishness of the Romans may be lost in the modern world, the potential uses of rose oil — the flower of love — remain as numerous today as in antiquity.

Sensuous Pleasures

Rose

A Relaxing, Harmonizing, and Arousing fragrance

Uses, Max. Drops

Bath oil, 3 in full bath

Facial oil, 2/1 Tbsp. base oil*

Body lotion, 3/1 Tbsp. base oil**

Perfume, 3–4/1 Tbsp. jojoba oil

Air fragrance, 3 in oil burner

Roughly one month's supply
**Equivalent to one handful of base oil*

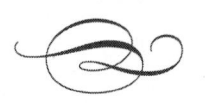

Rosemary

As Shakespeare's Ophelia said, mourning the loss of her father: "There's rosemary, that's for remembrance." Considered a sacred, almost magical plant since antiquity, rosemary was thought to stimulate the mind to remember and as such was used both to commemorate the dead and as an emblem of fidelity. As it revived memories and retrieved the past, so rosemary was said to restore the body to youthfulness. In some older versions of the fairy tale, Sleeping Beauty is awakened after a hundred years not by the kiss of a prince but by the smell of a sprig of rosemary. Rosemary was a key ingredient of "Hungary Water," a popular fourteenth-century toilet water that, according to legend, transformed the elderly and arthritic Queen of Hungary into such a beauty that she became the wife of the young King of Poland. The essential oil of rosemary is distilled from a vigorous evergreen shrub with ascending brown branches, stiff needlelike dark green leaves, and clusters of tiny pale blue flowers. According to Spanish tradition, the Virgin Mary is said to have spread her cloak over a rosemary bush, turning white flowers into blue, her symbolic color. Rosemary oil is perhaps the most stimulating of all the aromatic oils and is still used today, as in ancient Greece and Rome, to strengthen the mind, stimulate the body, and rejuvenate the appearance.

Fragrance

Herbal

Colorless to the palest yellow, rosemary oil has a clear, penetrating yet pleasing aroma that combines with other oils to create some of the loveliest perfumes, including the classic eau de cologne. A refreshing middle note, the fragrance blends especially well with black pepper, the citrus oils, cypress, frankincense, geranium, juniper, lavender, neroli, peppermint, rose, and thyme.

Effects on Mood and Emotion

Students in ancient Greece and Rome wore wreaths of rosemary around their heads to increase memory and concentration. Today rosemary oil continues to be used for these same reasons and is often the first choice of an aromatic oil to stimulate mental activity. An invigorating fragrance, rosemary restores clarity when there is mental fatigue and triggers the will to overcome obstacles such as inertia or indecision. As a strengthener, rosemary protects against negative emotions and provides support in times of stress.

Suggested Uses

An herbal published in 1525 claims: "Take thee a box of wood of rosemary and smell to it, and it shall preserve youth." While delightfully overstated here, rosemary oil is renowned as a restorative and rejuvenator, particularly for mature skin. The stimulating properties of rosemary extend to all spheres; the oil is thus a reliable energizer whether used in the bath, as a body lotion, an empowering perfume, or a fragrance in the air.

Caution

Avoid during pregnancy, or if there is a history of epilepsy or high blood pressure.

• • •

Oils to Enhance Clarity and Concentration

Basil

Black Pepper

Clove

Juniper

Lemon

Peppermint

Rosemary

Thyme

Sensuous Pleasures

Rosemary
An Uplifting and Stimulating fragrance

Uses, Max. Drops

Bath oil, 3–4 in full bath

Facial oil, 1/1 Tbsp. base oil*

Body lotion, 3–4/1 Tbsp. base oil**

Perfume, 5/1 Tbsp. jojoba oil

Air fragrance, 4 in oil burner

Roughly one month's supply
**Equivalent to one handful of base oil*

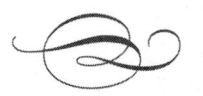

Sandalwood

Mentioned in the Nirukta, a Vedic religious text dating to the fifth century B.C., the sacred sandalwood tree of India has been burned as incense for thousands of years as a means of gaining access to the mystical. To Eastern religions what frankincense is to Western religions, the fragrance of the burning wood is said to quiet the mind and free the spirit, allowing for elevated, perhaps even ecstatic, states of consciousness. Sandalwood is still used in the East whether burned on the funeral pyre to liberate the soul of the deceased, inhaled as incense to aid meditation, or ground into paste and anointed on the foreheads of Hindu holy men as a mark of their spirituality. The essential oil of sandalwood, which has properties similar to its parent tree, is one of the oldest and most precious perfumes in the world. It is distilled from the now endangered sandalwood tree, whose wood built the temples of the East. This slender evergreen tree has brownish gray bark, smooth branches, leathery leaves, and pale yellow or purple flowers. Sandalwood is extremely slow growing, reaching full maturity after thirty years and living up to eighty years. Semiparasitic, it requires nourishment from the roots of a neighboring host tree for the first seven years of growth. Sandalwood trees are today protected by the Indian government, which runs an extensive propagation program. The tree is now cut down only when fully mature, and most of the wood is used for distillation of its beautifully exotic oil.

Fragrance
Woodland

A thick, pale to dark yellow oil, sandalwood has one of the most long-lasting aromas and is thus frequently used as a fixative in fine perfumes. The fragrance is rich, woody, and warm, with a sweet oriental undertone. A deep base note that is slightly masculine, sandalwood oil blends well with many fragrances, including black pepper, cedarwood, chamomile, the citrus oils, cypress, frankincense, geranium, jasmine, juniper, lavender, neroli, rose, vetivert, and ylang ylang.

Effects on Mood and Emotion

In several Eastern religions, the fragrance of sandalwood is used to awaken sexual energy so that it may be transformed into higher, more spiritual states of being. As an aphrodisiac, the oil restores natural inclination and increases the imagination when there is dullness or disinterest. As a stimulant to the creative urge, which is sexuality at its deepest root, the fragrance of sandalwood frees the mind from the mundane and may induce an almost euphoric state of awareness. In this place of heightened consciousness, sandalwood oil acts as an aid to meditation and encourages feelings of joy and acceptance. A primarily soothing scent, sandalwood may be used today to relieve stress, anxiety, and depression.

Suggested Uses

The inspiring, sensuously stirring scent of sandalwood is a beautiful addition to an evening bath, either to relax before a dream-filled sleep or to ready the heart for romance. The essence of enticement, the fragrance of sandalwood is the essence of perfume for body and soul.

Sensuous Pleasures

Sandalwood
A Relaxing and Arousing fragrance

Uses, Max. Drops

Bath oil, 5–6 in full bath

Facial oil, 3/1 Tbsp. base oil*

Body lotion, 6/1 Tbsp. base oil**

Perfume, 7/1 Tbsp. jojoba oil

Air fragrance, 4 in oil burner

Roughly one month's supply
**Equivalent to one handful of base oil*

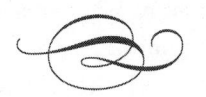

Thyme

Thought to be derived from the Greek *thumon*, meaning to burn a sacrifice, thyme was frequently used as incense on ancient temple altars probably because of the profound ability of the fragrance to focus the mind and strengthen the will. Thyme was believed by the Greeks to increase courage, and Roman soldiers bathed in it before going off to battle. During the Middle Ages, sprigs of thyme were sewn into the clothing of the Crusaders to promote bravery, or given to a jousting knight by his beloved. Indeed the essence derived from this common perennial herb is one of the most powerfully stimulating aromatic oils. On a mental level, the oil increases concentration, memory, and general mental acuity. On an emotional level, it revives the spirits and stimulates the desire to take decisive, positive action. There are many varieties of thyme: *Thymus vulgaris*, which has small gray-green oval leaves and tiny pink or lilac flowers, probably originates from *Thymus serpyllum* or wild thyme. Originally grown on the hillsides of Athens, wild thyme was taken to the rest of Europe by the Romans, where it became a popular culinary and medicinal herb. Numerous subspecies have since developed, each with its own particular chemical composition depending on climate, altitude, and other environmental variations. Rare among plants, thyme transplanted from one locale to another begins to exhibit characteristics endemic to the new site — testimony of the plant's versatility, adaptability, and capacity to successfully face challenges.

Fragrance

Herbal

A thick oil, thyme may be either reddish brown or clear with an aroma that is intense: hot, powerful, and penetrating. A distinctive middle note, thyme blends well with bergamot, grapefruit, lavender, lemon, melissa, and rosemary.

Effects on Mood and Emotion

The fragrance of thyme encourages the flow of vital energy to the mind and emotional centers. As such, it may be used to strengthen the memory, focus concentration, and overcome mental exhaustion, especially when due to anxiety or depression. Its powerful effect may also be seen on the will, where thyme oil is said to build initiative and the courage to act.

Suggested Uses

An invigorating oil, thyme is wonderful as an energizing morning bath oil, a refreshing foot soak, or a stimulating body rub. When vaporized into the atmosphere, the fragrance builds strength, vitality, and self-confidence.

Caution

Avoid during pregnancy, or if there is a history of high blood pressure or overactive thyroid. Use as recommended to prevent possible tingling or irritation of the skin.

Thyme
A Stimulating fragrance

Uses, Max. Drops

Bath oil, 3 in full bath

Body lotion, 3/1 Tbsp. base oil*

Perfume, 2–3/1 Tbsp. jojoba oil

Air fragrance, 3 in oil burner

Equivalent to one handful of base oil

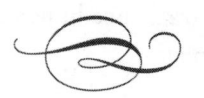

Vetivert

Vetivert is a tall, wild aromatic grass that thrives in the warm, moist soil of the tropics from the Caribbean Islands to Tahiti. The grass is frequently woven into mats, shades, or thatched roofs, and after a summer storm it gives off an exquisite scent that perfumes the air. Vetivert oil is distilled from the strong reddish roots of this perennial grass that are dug out by hand, then cleaned, dried in the sun, cut into fine pieces, and soaked in water prior to steam distillation. Called "the oil of tranquility," vetivert has a rich aroma that is protecting and grounding. The oil is reputed to instill feelings of safety based on a firm connection with reality and the intention to live life according to the highest ideals.

Fragrance

Musky

A very thick, dark amber to deep reddish-brown oil, vetivert has a woody, warm, musky, and distinctly earthy aroma. The oil is an excellent fixative in perfumes and is a main component of many beautiful scents, especially in the Orient. As a penetrating base note, vetivert oil blends well with frankincense, geranium, jasmine, neroli, orange, rose, sandalwood, and ylang ylang.

Effects on Mood and Emotion

Due to its deeply relaxing and calming properties, the fragrance of vetivert is highly beneficial for relieving extreme anxiety, nervous tension, and resultant insomnia. Used in folk magic for protection, the oil guards against injury through oversensitivity, strengthens inner determination, and engenders a spirit of acceptance and forgiveness. With its earthy scent, vetivert evokes a physical sensuality and is a renowned aphrodisiac, especially in the East.

Suggested Uses

Vetivert oil is a revitalizing tonic that helps bring back a silky softness to mature skin. The tranquil yet sensually inspiring fragrance also makes a lovely addition to a nighttime bath or an exotic body rub. As a perfume or essence in the air, vetivert conveys a safe, enveloping sense of stillness.

Sensuous Pleasures

Vetivert.

A Relaxing and Arousing fragrance

Uses, Max. Drops

Bath oil, 1–2 in full bath

Facial oil, 1/1 Tbsp. base oil*

Body lotion, 2/1 Tbsp. base oil**

Perfume, 4/1 Tbsp. jojoba oil

Air fragrance, 1–2 in oil burner

Roughly one month's supply
**Equivalent to one handful of base oil*

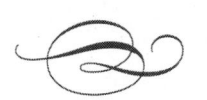

Ylang Ylang

The luxuriousness of the tropics is evoked by the fragrance of ylang ylang (pronounced "ee-lang ee-lang"), the flower of the "perfume tree." This semiwild tree has a brittle bark and shiny oval leaves with unusually large mauve or yellow flowers. The yellow flowers have the sweetest, most voluptuous scent and produce the finest oil. In the South Seas, women rub ylang ylang mixed with cucuma flowers and coconut oil—a concoction called "borri-borri"—on their skin and hair to add softness, shine, and fragrance. The beneficial effects of ylang ylang on hair growth made it a key ingredient of the nineteenth-century hair care preparation known as Macassar Oil. This became so popular that the Victorians had to protect their chair backs against greasy hair stains with "anti-macassars." The essential oil of ylang ylang captures the sensuality of this flower of flowers for total aesthetic pleasure, from perfumed bathing to erotic massage.

Fragrance

Floral

The light yellow syrupy oil of ylang ylang is intensely sweet, and perhaps most effective when combined with other essences that lighten its fragrance. This lingering oil makes an excellent base note in perfumes and blends well with numerous other fragrances including black pepper, the citrus oils, frankincense, jasmine, lavender, patchouli, rose, and sandalwood.

Effects on Mood and Emotion

The evocative fragrance of ylang ylang is one of the most reliable aromatic aphrodisiacs. It is said to awaken a voluptuousness that craves release, as well as an open, generous giving of the self to another. The fragrance of ylang ylang lifts and calms the emotions, creating a balanced, mellow mood where anger, frustration, fear, and sadness are soothed away.

Suggested Uses

The exotic scent of ylang ylang sets a mellow mood for relaxation and pleasure whether used in the bath, as a body rub, perfume, or essence in the air. The oil has a toning and balancing effect on the skin, making it beneficial for dry or oily as well as mature skin. As a natural hair tonic, ylang ylang is one of the loveliest aromatic oils to fragrance the hair while adding gloss and body.

Caution

Use in low concentrations as recommended to prevent possible headache or nausea.

Sensuous Pleasures

Ylang Ylang
A Relaxing and Arousing fragrance

Uses, Max. Drops

Bath oil, 3–4 in full bath

Facial oil, 2/1 Tbsp. base oil*

Body lotion, 4/1 Tbsp. base oil**

Perfume, 8/1 Tbsp. jojoba oil

Air fragrance, 3 in oil burner

Roughly one month's supply
**Equivalent to one handful of base oil*

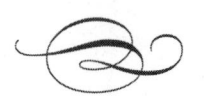

Base Oils

The essential oils must always be diluted
in a carrier or base oil that is extracted
from the flesh, nut, or seeds of plants.
Unlike the essential oils, these plant oils
leave an oily residue on the skin and their
odor does not evaporate (i.e., the scent is
"fixed"). As they comprise the greatest
proportion of an aromatic blend, and as
each plant oil has its own nutritional constituents and characteristics, this guide
outlines the most suitable base oils for a
particular use or mode of application.

• • •

Avocado Oil

Texture: Thick, heavy

Permeability: Easily absorbed

Properties: Soothes and softens dry, dehydrated skin; revitalizes and regenerates mature skin

First used by the Aztec Indians as a food and an aphrodisiac, avocado oil has long been a traditional beauty oil among the native people of Mexico and Arizona. The avocado tree is indigenous to the swamplands of South America and is still called "alligator pear" by some. A distant relative of the fragrant magnolia tree, avocado was one of the first vegetable oils to be used in beauty care, probably because it is so easily extracted from the flesh of the fruit. The oil of the avocado fruit is thick, heavy and, if unrefined, a dark emerald green. Despite its viscosity, avocado oil is easily absorbed and penetrates deeply into the skin. Because of its high vitamin A and E content, the oil is especially useful to soothe and soften dry, dehydrated skin, as well as to help revitalize and regenerate mature skin. Although expensive, especially if unrefined, avocado oil can be effectively combined with other base oils, such as sweet almond, to create a less costly yet still nourishing blend.

Grapeseed Oil

Texture: Very light and non-greasy

Permeability: Easily absorbed

Properties: Slightly astringent

As its name implies, this plant oil is extracted from the seeds of grapes, most of which originate in the vineyards of France. While the grape is an ancient fruit, extraction of the 6–20 percent oil content from its seeds is a relatively new process. The particular advantage of grapeseed as a base oil lies in its extremely light and non-greasy texture that, combined with its easy absorbability, makes it an excellent choice for whole-body massage blends. As it is slightly astringent, the oil may also be particularly useful for oily skin. Almost colorless or a pale yellowish-green, grapeseed oil is odorless and will not interfere with the delicate scents of the essential oils. If desired, it may be combined with more nutritious albeit more expensive plant oils, such as avocado oil.

Hazelnut Oil

Texture: Light

Permeability: Easily absorbed

Properties: Slightly astringent

It is reported that hazelnut oil was first extracted from the small kernels of the hazelnut tree during the Bronze Age, making it one of the oldest plant oils in existence. Today the nuts, which are also called filberts or cobnuts, may be found growing on tall treelike shrubs throughout Europe, although most hazelnut oil now comes from Southern France. Here the oil is left to settle in large vats for a week or so until the sediment has sunk to the bottom, and then it is filtered by hand. A lovely amber yellow with a subtle nutty aroma, hazelnut oil is light and more easily absorbed than most plant oils, and is thus an excellent base oil for face and body massage blends. As it is one of the more expensive plant oils, hazelnut may be combined with grapeseed oil, which is far less costly.

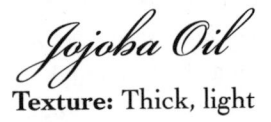

Jojoba Oil

Texture: Thick, light

Permeability: Easily absorbed

Properties: Richly moisturizing for all skin types; thickens and beautifies hair

Pronounced "ho-ho-ba," this versatile oil comes from a desert plant indigenous to South America, and is now found primarily in northern Mexico and the southwestern United States. A hardy evergreen shrub with gray-green leaves and small brown nuts, jojoba thrives in arid desert soil due to its thirteen-foot root system, and is not surprisingly one of nature's finest sources of moisture. Jojoba nuts ripen throughout the summer and fall to the ground in autumn, at which time the oil may be extracted from the pod seeds. The extracted oil is actually not an oil per se, but a liquid wax; in fact, jojoba has the distinction of being the only plant to contain a liquid wax.

Also known as deer nut, wild hazel, coffee berry, and goat nut, jojoba was classified by the English botanist H. F. Link in the 1840s but already had been a favorite of native North Americans for centuries. Traditionally the oil was applied externally to help heal wounds and sores, or was taken internally for the relief of stomach ailments and eye, throat, and skin infections. However, the popular modern use of jojoba oil was widely developed only during the 1970s as an alternative to sperm whale oil. Like spermaceti, the waxy substance derived from the head of the sperm whale, jojoba oil adds thickness to cosmetic preparations and is similarly effective in soothing, softening, and moisturizing the skin.

The pale golden yellow oil of jojoba has a light, fine texture that penetrates deeply into the skin — more deeply than most other plant oils. This, combined with its long shelf life, makes jojoba an ideal base for the essential oils. When dotted on the skin as perfume or used as a lubricating and nourishing face or body lotion, the odorless, easily spreadable jojoba adds a silky luxuriousness to any blend. Jojoba was renowned among the native people of Mexico and Arizona for its ability to add sheen and luster to the hair and is still recommended as a thickening tonic for the hair.

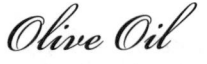

Olive Oil

Texture: Thick, slightly sticky

Permeability: Easily absorbed

Properties: Soothes and moisturizes dry dehydrated skin; thickens and beautifies hair

Although it takes up to ten years for an olive tree to bear fruit, the tree can flourish for centuries and was considered a symbol of strength and fertility by many ancient civilizations. The Egyptians and Greeks believed the olive tree was a gift from the gods; in the Old Testament, Moses is instructed by the Lord to prepare a holy anointing oil consisting of myrrh, sweet cinnamon, calamus, cassia, and olive oil. Just as the olive tree was regarded as a divine gift, so too it was used by man as an offering of friendship, forgiveness, and peace—a concept still existing today. The Greeks, whose landscape was abundant with olive trees, valued the oil as currency, food, fuel, medicine, and cosmetic, and indeed olive oil is one of the oldest beauty care ingredients.

A natural source of vitamin E, the oil is especially valuable in aromatic blends to soothe and nourish the skin or to moisturize dry, dehydrated skin. The Egyptians and Greeks rubbed olive oil in their hair and it is still recommended to increase both body and shine. Olive oil is very easily obtained and is one of the longest lasting plant oils, especially if kept away from light and heat. A little heavy, with a strong odor, this wonderfully soothing ancient oil may be combined with a lighter, odorless oil such as grapeseed.

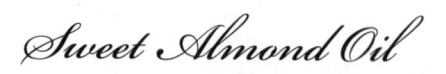

Sweet Almond Oil

Texture: Slides easily

Permeability: Easily absorbed

Properties: Softens and soothes the skin; heals rough hands and strengthens nails

The sweet almond tree is a native of the eastern Mediterranean and its history can be traced back to biblical times. The rod of Aaron is reputed to have been a branch of the almond tree, although its symbolism is lost to present generations. This lovely tree, which belongs to the same botanical family as the peach and apricot, has delicate pinky-white blossoms that flower in January. The almonds form on short branches and are encased in a thick gray husk that opens when the nut is ready. The tree was a favorite of the Romans, who planted it along the routes of their European conquests.

The oil is pale yellow with an almost odorless, slightly nutty aroma. It penetrates deeply and slides easily and is therefore an excellent base oil for face and body massage blends. Sweet almond oil is beneficial for all skin types, but particularly for softening dry, sensitive skin or for calming irritated and sore skin on the body, face, or hands. The sixteenth-century British herbalist John Gerard wrote that almond oil "makes smoothe thye hands and face," and "creme amande" was a popular moisturizer and hand cream in the court of Napoleon and Josephine. Sweet almond oil has a fairly long shelf life and is less expensive than many other plant oils. It may be combined with lighter oils such as grapeseed or with more expensive oils such as jojoba or avocado for a truly luxurious aromatic blend.

To Obtain the Fragrances

Pure essential oils, while more expensive than adulterated or synthetic fragrances, have the loveliest aromas and offer the greatest potential benefits. These natural fragrances are widely available through local suppliers, by mail order, or via the Internet. Some suggestions follow.

Local Sources

Health-food stores

Beauty clinics & spas

Speciality fragrance & perfume shops

Herbal apothecaries

New Age suppliers

Mail Order and Internet Suppliers

AromaCare International Inc.

26 Chumleigh Crescent

Markham, Ontario L3T 4G6

Canada

Tel: 905-709-5754

Fax: 905-764-8043

e-mail: alam@aromacare.com

website: aromacare.com

(mail order)

Aromaland, Inc.
1326 Rufina Circle
Santa Fe, New Mexico 87505
Tel: 800-933-5267 (toll free)
Fax: 505-438-7223
e-mail: info@aromaland.com
website: aromaland.com
(online ordering)

Aroma Thyme
Tel: 888 AROMA 99 (toll free)
e-mail: sales@aromathyme.com
website: aromathyme.com
(online ordering)

Ashbury's Aromatherapy
145-3751 Jacombs Road
Richmond, British Columbia V6V 2RF
Canada
Tel: 604-276-9774
Fax: 604-276-9775
e-mail: michaels@ashburys.com
website: ashburys.com
(mail order and online ordering)

Bella House of Beauty
9020-C Beverly Blvd.
West Hollywood, California 90048
Tel: 310-859-1006
Fax: 818-576-8175
e-mail: sales@bellabeauty.com
website: bellabeauty.com
(mail order and online ordering)

Birch Hill Happenings
2898 County Road 103
Barnum, Minnesota 55707-8808
Tel: 218-384-9294
Fax: 218-384-3975
e-mail: albuddy@aol.com
website: birchhillhappenings.com
(mail order and online ordering)

Botanical Pleasures
Denver, Colorado
e-mail: botanicalpleasures@juno.com
website: botanicalpleasures.com
(online ordering)

Dreaming Earth Botanicals
P.O. Box 727
Penrose, North Carolina 28766
Tel/fax: 800-897-8330
e-mail: Info@dreamingearth.com
website: dreamingearth.com
(mail order and online ordering)

Gritman Essential Oils
P.O. Box 2009
Friendswood, Texas 77549
Tel: 888-GRITMAN (toll free), 281-996-0103
Fax: 281-996-0318
e-mail: shehad@gritman.com
website: gritman.com
(online ordering)

Helios Essential Oils
P.O. Box 561
Wheat Ridge, Colorado 80033
Tel: 888-327-9954 or 303-420-7172
Fax: 303-463-6224
e-mail: info@heliosoils.com
website: heliosoils.com
(online ordering)

J. Crow Company
P.O. Box 172
New Ipswich, New Hampshire 03071
Tel/fax: 800-878-1965 (toll free)
e-mail: jcrow@jcrows.mv.com
website: jcrows.com
(mail order and online ordering)

Leyden House, Limited
200 Brattelboro Road
Leyden, Massachusetts 01337
Tel: 800-754-0668
Fax: 413-772-8858
e-mail: leydeneo@javanet.com
website: leydenhouse.com
(mail order and online ordering)

Nature's Gift
1040 Cheyenne Blvd.
Madison, Tennessee 37115
Fax: 615-860-9171
e-mail: orderdesk@naturesgift.com
website: naturesgift.com
(online ordering)

One Planet
10247 East Covington Street
Tucson, Arizona 85748
Tel: 877-259-6392 (toll free)
Fax: 520-885-2487
e-mail: oneplanet@oneplanetnatural.com
website: oneplanetnatural.com
(mail order and online ordering)

Orysi
20 South Court Street
Thunder Bay, Ontario P7B 2W3
Canada
Tel: 807-345-4288
Fax: 807-345-2674
e-mail: emailus@orysi.com
website: orysi.com
(mail order and online ordering)

Snowdrift Farm Natural Products Inc.
P.O. Box 958
Jefferson, Maine 04348-0958
Tel: 888-999-6950 (toll free)
Fax: 207-549-4717
e-mail: info@snowdriftfarm.com
website: snowdriftfarm.com
(mail order and online ordering)

Torling Fragrance Products
8320 Cutler Way
Sacramento, California 95828
Tel/fax: 916-682-1334
e-mail: torset@jps.net
website: torlingfragrances.com
(mail order and online ordering)

Well, Naturally Products Ltd.
12706-114-A Avenue
Surrey, British Columbia V3V 3P4
Canada
Tel: 604-580-3468
Fax: 604-580-9548
e-mail: mary@wellnaturally.com
website: wellnaturally.com
(mail order)

Glossary

Aphrodisiac — Named after Aphrodite, Greek goddess of love, an aphrodisiac increases sexual desire or enjoyment.

Arousing — Used here as a category to describe those essential oils that stir feelings of love and desire.

Astringent — A substance that causes the skin to dry and tighten; usually associated with its capacity to cleanse and constrict the pores in oily skin.

Base note — In describing the volatility of an essential oil, base notes are those heavier fragrances that evaporate most slowly, and therefore have the most lingering aroma.

Base oil — Any vegetable or plant oil, such as grapeseed oil, sweet almond oil, or jojoba, that is used as a medium for the essential oils. Base oils, unlike essential oils, are non-volatile — their scent does not evaporate into the air.

Essence — The highly volatile fragrance of an aromatic plant, the essence is produced and stored in tiny oil glands located on the surface of a leaf, in the petals of the flower, the peel of a fruit, the roots, the resin, or the heartwood of a tree.

Essential oils — The extracted essence of an aromatic plant, essential oils are most commonly obtained via steam distillation, a process developed in the eleventh century to capture and transform ethereal fragrance into an essential oil.

Fixed oils — Unlike essential oils that are highly volatile and readily evaporate into the atmosphere, fixed oils are non-volatile; their fragrance is "fixed" and not fleeting.

Harmonizing — Used here as a category to describe those essential oils that balance the system, either relaxing or uplifting depending on need, but overall resulting in equilibrium and harmony.

Holism/holistic — The concept of "wholeness" or "oneness," holism considers man a complete entity of body, mind, emotion, and spirit. Holistic, therefore, implies uniformity or action as one unit.

Middle note — In describing the volatility of an essential oil, middle notes are those fragrances that evaporate at a moderate speed; middle notes generally form the "heart" or central core of a fragrant blend.

Pheromones — An individual's natural, distinctive odor; in the animal world, pheromones are used for recognition, marking territory, signaling danger, and attracting a mate.

Photosensitivity — Increased sensitivity to the sun or other sources of ultraviolet light. Some essential oils — primarily the citrus oils — cause photosensitivity and should thus be avoided before exposure to direct sunlight.

Relaxing—Used here as a category to describe those essential oils that are mentally and physically calming.

Stimulating—Used here as a category to describe those essential oils that are mentally stimulating—sharpening concentration, clear thinking, and memory—as well as physically energizing.

Synthetic—Not natural and artificial, synthetic fragrances are chemical reproductions of the pure fragrances that occur in nature.

Toners—Stimulating the circulation and reducing oiliness, toners refresh and rebalance the skin for healthy functioning; usually applied after cleansing.

Top note—In describing the volatility of an essential oil, top notes are those lighter fragrances that evaporate most quickly; top notes are the scent first noticed in a fragrant blend.

Unguent—An old-fashioned term to describe an ointment or salve, usually used in relation to beauty preparations.

Uplifting—Used here as a category to describe those essential oils that are emotionally uplifting and mood elevating.

Volatility—The volatility of an oil describes its capacity to freely and rapidly diffuse or evaporate into the atmosphere.

Bibliography

Ackerman, D. *A Natural History of the Senses*. New York: Random House, 1990.

Arcier, M. *Aromatherapy*. London: Reed International Books Ltd., 1992.

Bown, D. *The Royal Horticultural Society Encyclopedia of Herbs and Their Uses*. London: Dorling Kindersley Ltd., 1995.

Bremness, L. *Herbs Eyewitness Handbooks*. London: Dorling Kindersley Ltd., 1994.

Brown, D. *Aromatherapy*. London: Headway Lifeguides (Hodder and Stoughton), 1993.

Chinery, M. *Field Guide to the Plant Life of Britain and Europe*. London: Kingfisher Books Ltd. (A Grisewood and Dempsey Company), 1987.

Cunningham, S. *Magical Aromatherapy — The Power of Scent*. St. Paul, Minnesota: Llewellyn Publications, 1989.

Davis, P. *Subtle Aromatherapy*. London: The C. W. Daniel Company Ltd., 1991.

Drury, N. and S. Drury. *Healing Oils and Essences*. London: Robert Hale Ltd., 1988.

Flück, H. *Medicinal Plants*. Hong Kong: W. Foulsham and Co. Ltd., 1988.

Guenther, E. *The Essential Oils*. London: Van Nostrand Co. (Reinhold), 1948.

Hopkins, C. *The Joy of Aromatherapy — Sensual Remedies for Everyday Ailments*. London: Angus and Robertson (HarperCollins Publishers), 1991.

Keeler, E. *Aromatherapy Handbook for Beauty, Hair, and Skin Care*. Vermont: Healing Arts Press, 1991.

Lavabre, M. *Aromatherapy Workbook*. Vermont: Healing Arts Press, Inner Traditions, Inc., 1990.

Lawless, J. *Home Aromatherapy — Guide to Using Essential Oils at Home*. London: Kyle Cathie, 1995.

Lee, W. and L. Lee. *The Book of Practical Aromatherapy.* San Francisco: Keats Publishing Inc., 1992.

Le Guérer, A. *Scent—The Essential and Mysterious Powers of Smell.* New York: Kodansha International, 1994.

Maury, M. *Marguerite Maury's Guide to Aromatherapy—The Secret of Life and Youth.* London: The C.W. Daniel Company Ltd., 1989.

Press, B. *Herbs Green Guide.* London: New Holland (Publishers Ltd.), 1994.

Price, S. *Aromatherapy Workbook.* London: Thorsons (HarperCollins Publishers), 1993.

Sellar, W. *The Directory of Essential Oils.* London: The C. W. Daniel Company Ltd.,1992.

Tisserand, M. *Aromatherapy for Lovers.* London: Thorsons (HarperCollins Publishers Ltd.), 1993.

———. *Aromatherapy for Women.* London: Thorsons (HarperCollins Publishers Ltd.), 1985.

———. *The 14-Day Aromabeauty Plan—How to Look Better, Feel Better in Two Aromatic Weeks.* London: Vermilion (Random House), 1994.

Tisserand, R. *The Art of Aromatherapy.* London: The C.W. Daniel Company Ltd., 1977.

Valnet, J. *The Practice of Aromatherapy.* London: The C. W. Daniel Company Ltd., 1980.

Vroon, P. *Smell, The Secret Seducer.* New York: Farrar, Straus and Giroux, 1994.

Wildwood, C. *Creative Aromatherapy.* London: Thorsons (HarperCollins Publishers Ltd.), 1993.

Winter, R. *The Smell Book—Scents, Sex, and Society.* New York: J. B. Lippincott Company, 1976.

Worwood, V. A. *Aromatics—Romance, Love, Sex, and Nature's Essential Oils.* Canada: Bantam Books, 1987.

———. *The Fragrant Pharmacy—A Home Health Care Guide to Aromatherapy and Essential Oils.* London: Macmillan London Ltd., 1990.

Index

REACH FOR THE MOON

Llewellyn publishes hundreds of books on your favorite subjects! To get these exciting books, including the one on the following page, check your local bookstore or order them directly from Llewellyn.

ORDER BY PHONE

- Call toll-free within the U.S. and Canada, 1-800-THE MOON
- In Minnesota, call (651) 291-1970
- We accept VISA, MasterCard, and American Express

ORDER BY MAIL

- Send the full price of your order (MN residents add 7% sales tax) in U.S. funds, plus postage & handling to:

Llewellyn Worldwide
P.O. Box 64383, Dept. 1-56718-491-X
St. Paul, MN 55164-0383, USA

POSTAGE & HANDLING

(For the U.S., Canada, and Mexico)
- $4.00 for orders $15.00 and under
- $5.00 for orders over $15.00
- No charge for orders over $100.00

We ship UPS in the continental United States. We ship standard mail to P.O. boxes. Orders shipped to Alaska, Hawaii, the Virgin Islands, and Puerto Rico are sent first-class mail. Orders shipped to Canada and Mexico are sent surface mail.

International orders: Airmail—add freight equal to price of each book to the total price of order, plus $5.00 for each non-book item (audio tapes, etc.). Surface mail—Add $1.00 per item.

Allow 2 weeks for delivery on all orders. Postage and handling rates subject to change.

DISCOUNTS

We offer a 20% discount to group leaders or agents. You must order a minimum of 5 copies of the same book to get our special quantity price.

FREE CATALOG

Get a free copy of our color catalog, *New Worlds of Mind and Spirit*. Subscribe for just $10.00 in the United States and Canada ($30.00 overseas, airmail). Many bookstores carry *New Worlds*—ask for it!

Visit our website at www.llewellyn.com for more information.

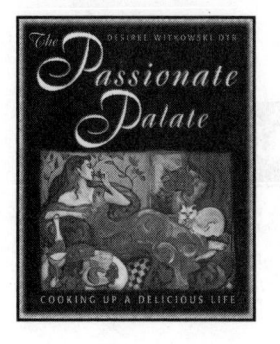

The Passionate Palate
Recipes for Cooking Up a Delicious Life

DESIRÉE WITKOWSKI, D.T.R.

Soothe your soul with a heavenly bowl of mashed potatoes, cool off on a hot July afternoon with a Sangria of the Gods, and remember that passionate kissing burns 6.4 calories a minute.

For emotional health, women actually require a minimum of one hour every day of something that feels good. Indulge all five senses, then move onto your sense of daring, your sense of romance, and your sense of humor. Watch yourself come alive when you choose to validate yourself and reclaim the quiet times (or hell-raising times) that you need.

Based on Jungian psychology, *The Passionate Palate* is a hybrid self-help/personal essay/cookbook—a 40/60 ration of easy-to-make comfort foods laced with practical tips, meditations, and inspirational quotations to guide women toward de-stressing life and finding their innate power.

Whether or not you like to cook or even know how, *The Passionate Palate* will leave you feeling warm, full, and contented, with old-fashioned recipes and new-fashioned ways to pamper your psyche and spirit.

1-56718-824-9
480 pp., 7½ x 9⅛, 2-color   **$21.95**

To order, call 1-800-THE MOON
Prices subject to change without notice